Teaching Memory to Adults

Includes the complete text of

Improving Your Memory

How to Remember What You're Starting to Forget

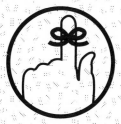

Janet Fogler and Lynn Stern

REVISED EDITION

Teaching Memory Improvement to Adults

REVISED EDITION

Janet Fogler, M.S.W.

and

Lynn Stern, M.S.W.

The Johns Hopkins University Press

Baltimore and London

We would like to express our appreciation and gratitude to the
W. K. Kellogg Foundation and to all of our colleagues at the
Turner Geriatric Clinic, especially Ruth Campbell. We are also
indebted to Bea Wolley and to all of the Turner Peer Counselors
who began the memory program in 1978. Lastly, we want to thank
Scott and Neal for their good humor and support.

© 1987 Janet Fogler and Lynn Stern
© 1994 The Johns Hopkins University Press
All rights reserved. Published 1994.
Printed in the United States of America on acid-free paper
03 02 01 00 99 98 97 96 95 94   5 4 3 2 1

The Johns Hopkins University Press
2715 North Charles Street
Baltimore, Maryland 21218-4319
The Johns Hopkins Press Ltd., London

ISBN 0-8018-4769-9 (pbk).

Library of Congress Cataloging-in-Publication Data will be found at the end of this book.

A catalog record for this book is available from the British Library.

The complete text of *Improving Your Memory: How to Remember What You're Starting to Forget* follows in boxed pages—like this one.

Contents

Preface   ix

1. **How Memory Works   1**

2. **How Memory Changes as People Age   17**

3. **Factors Affecting Memory for People of All Ages   27**

4. **Memory Improvement Techniques   59**

   General Tips for Remembering   91

   Answers to the Exercises   95

   Recommended Reading   99

Contents

Preface   vii

The complete text of the student workbook,
Improving Your Memory: How to Remember What You're Starting to Forget   1

    Accompanied throughout by:

    Introductions

    Additional examples and exercises

    Notes to the teacher

    And other supplementary material

Review Exercises   95

How to Offer a Memory Course   99

Recommended Reading   107

Improving Your Memory
Preface

If you frequently say, "I just can't remember anymore!" or "My memory has gotten *so* bad!" you may have given in to the myth that aging and memory loss go hand in hand. In fact, it is the belief in this myth that keeps many people from even *trying* to remember. People of all ages complain about forgetting, but older people often worry about getting "senile" when they cannot remember a cousin's name or where they put their appointment book. There *are* changes in memory as people grow older, but, for almost everyone, memory can be improved with training and practice.

No one can remember everything. People of all ages must make choices about what they want to remember and put effort and energy into those areas that are most important to them. This self-help manual will enable you to make these choices, based on an understanding of how memory works and how it changes with age, and will give you concrete strategies for tackling the areas of memory that trouble you.

In order to make the basic information more meaningful, we have included many examples from everyday life, pen-and-paper exercises demonstrating concepts and techniques, and assignments for applying what you have learned to your daily life.

You will get the most out of this book if you read it carefully, do all of the exercises, and make an effort to use the suggestions in your daily life.

Preface

As clinical social workers in an outpatient medical setting for people over sixty, we became increasingly aware of the deep concerns of older people about memory. Our patients wondered about the significance of being unable to find the car in the parking lot or letting the pot boil over one more time. The belief in inevitable "senility" and the fear of its onset were pervasive.

In response to the demand for information about memory and aging, we decided to create a comprehensive, concise, and accessible memory program for older adults. The literature on aging and memory is vast, and our task has been to extract and interpret the information that is most relevant to memory improvement for older people. Through many years of experimentation, we developed a memory course with a format that proved to be both meaningful and fun. Under a grant from the W. K. Kellogg Foundation, we were funded to train other professionals to replicate the course in their own settings. We developed a training manual for this purpose. At the same time, we recognized that there were many older adults who would not have access to a memory course. Thus, we developed a book that could be used as a self-paced guidebook as well as a text for a memory course.

How to Use This Manual

In the first section of this manual, we have combined notes to the teacher, supplementary material, and additional examples with a replica of the student text, *Improving Your Memory: How to Remember What You're Starting to Forget.* We have found the course to be most effective when each student has his or her own copy of the student text for between-class reading and assignments. Because the use of examples is a very effective teaching tool, we have included new examples that are not part of the student guide for your use in class presentations. At the end of the first section, you will find a review exercise that synthesizes the information on memory improvement techniques and can be used as a trigger for problem-solving.

Although you can offer a memory course using only this book and the accompanying student text, we encourage you to expand your knowledge about the memory process before you begin teaching memory improvement to other people. You may find it helpful to refer to some of the books listed in "Recommended Reading" at the end of this book and spend some time thinking about memory. The more you learn about memory, the better teacher you will be.

In the second section of this manual, you'll find information on "How to Offer a Memory Course." Included are course objectives, a description of the course format that we have found most successful, and information on publicity and evaluation. Also included is a sample agenda for a four-session memory course. An important part of the memory course is group discussion and support, so if you find that you can't present all of the information in the stated time frame, we suggest that you extend the number of sessions rather than eliminate the opportunity for group discussion and sharing of experiences.

The complete text of the student workbook *Improving Your Memory: How to Remember What You're Starting to Forget,* accompanied throughout by introductions, additional examples and exercises, notes to the teacher, and other supplementary material

1   How Memory Works

To improve the memory process, it helps to understand how memory works. Although the brain is not understood nearly as well as the heart or the circulatory system, memory experts have devised a way to visualize how we remember. They often describe the memory process as consisting of three stages.

The Three Stages of Memory

Sensory memory, the first stage in the memory process, is the very brief recognition by the mind of what the senses take in. We become aware of information through the senses—vision, hearing, touch, smell, and taste. In the world in which we live, we are constantly surrounded by sights and sounds. Much of what the eye sees and the ear hears is discarded immediately. There is no need for us to record it. However, when the sensory impression is paid attention to, it enters the second stage of memory, known as short-term memory.

Short-term memory may be equated with conscious thought—the very small amount of material that you can hold in your mind at any one moment. Most experts believe that short-term memory can hold no more than six or seven items. This material will be forgotten in five to ten seconds, unless it is continually repeated or it is transferred to long-term memory.

When working with older adults, it is a challenge to describe a model for how memory works in a way that is easily understood and relevant to their interests and goals. When we first developed a memory course for older adults, we put little emphasis on the memory process, but we now recognize that a basic understanding of how memory works is the foundation of memory improvement. If you don't know the basics of how a car works, you can't fix it.

An understanding of how memory works provides a framework for understanding why things are either remembered or forgotten. Students can use this information to analyze their own memory failures and to determine what went wrong in the process. Throughout the course, additional information, such as factors that affect memory and memory improvement techniques, will be related to the stages of the memory process.

An example of information that is held in short-term memory and generally discarded without being stored is a seven-digit telephone number. When you look up a phone number, close the phone book, dial the number, and get a busy signal, you often realize that you've already forgotten the number you just dialed. This is a good demonstration of how briefly information is held in short-term memory. *It is important to keep in mind that not all information that registers in short-term memory gets stored in long-term memory.*

Long-term memory, the memory bank, is the largest component of the memory system. Its storage space is practically limitless. A common misconception is that long-term memory refers to events that occurred a long time ago. In fact, long-term memory holds information that was learned as recently as a few minutes ago and as long ago as many decades. This storage space holds items as varied as:

- your name

- what happened an hour ago

- where you spent last Thanksgiving

- the information needed to drive a car

- the image of your first-grade teacher

- the multiplication tables

Thus, long-term memory refers to any information that is no longer in conscious thought but is stored for potential recollection.

The diagram on page 3 summarizes the memory process, which is more fully explained on the following pages.

Supplementary Material *(The Three Stages of Memory)*

The brain is not as well understood as many other parts of the body. Although we describe a well-defined three-stage model for how memory works, future research may give us a different depiction of the memory process. In your reading you may find that some authors have chosen to talk about how memory works by using a four-stage model. We decided to base our course on a three-stage model because it is easily understood and relevant to the objectives of the course.

Note to the Teacher *(The Three Stages of Memory)*

It is very important for students to understand the difference between our working definitions of short- and long-term memory (see *Improving Your Memory,* p. 1–2). Just because something is registered in short-term memory (conscious thought) does not mean it has been stored in long-term memory and is available for recall at a later time. For example, a person may hear a statistic on the radio, be amazed at the meaning of it, and later be totally unable to recall or even recognize the exact number. When your students say "I forgot," ask them to analyze the situation and consider the possibility that the information never made it into long-term memory.

Supplementary Material *(The Three Stages of Memory)*

Even though we have presented the stages of memory as if information entered each stage in consecutive order, it is possible for information that has not registered in conscious thought to be stored in long-term memory. There are situations in which people remember things without being aware of them. For example, you may not be consciously aware of all of the people sitting in the doctor's waiting room with you, but when a man comes in and asks if you have seen a woman in a wheelchair, you recall that the nurse took a woman in a wheelchair into an exam room.

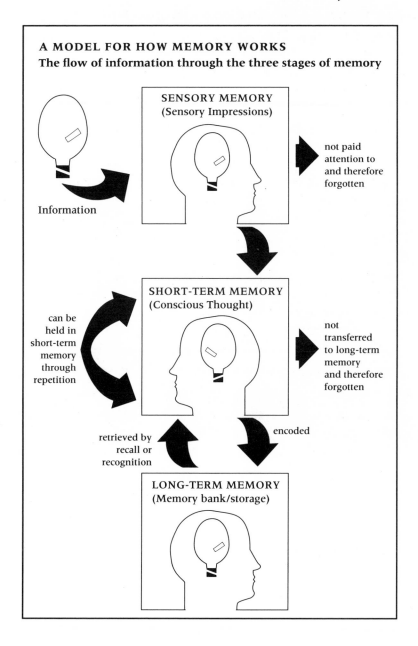

A MODEL FOR HOW MEMORY WORKS
The flow of information through the three stages of memory

SENSORY MEMORY
(Sensory Impressions)

not paid attention to and therefore forgotten

Information

can be held in short-term memory through repetition

SHORT-TERM MEMORY
(Conscious Thought)

not transferred to long-term memory and therefore forgotten

retrieved by recall or recognition

encoded

LONG-TERM MEMORY
(Memory bank/storage)

Additional Example *(The Three Stages of Memory)*

You are addressing envelopes containing announcements of the church bazaar. You have a list of names but no addresses. Your task is to look up the names in the phone book and transfer the addresses to the envelopes. As you handle the phone book, your senses take in the feel of the book, the faint smell of the ink, the pattern of the names on a given page, the sound of pages turning. However, these sensory impressions may or may not register in conscious thought.

You find Florence Tillman's name in the phone book and copy her address onto an envelope, 4276 Woodlawn, Chelsea, Michigan. This information has entered short-term memory. You can hold it in mind for the few seconds needed to address the envelope. If you are not familiar with this street, you are unlikely to store this information in long-term memory. After a few moments, you probably won't even remember the name of the street.

However, if you note that Woodlawn Street is in your sister's neighborhood and you wonder if she knows Ms. Tillman, you are more likely to transfer the information to long-term memory and think of Ms. Tillman as you drive down Woodlawn on the way to your sister's house.

Here is an example of how the memory process works in daily life.

EXAMPLE

- You are doing your weekly shopping at the local grocery store. There are many items on the shelves which make sensory impressions on you. You see the colors of the packages, smell the bakery products, and hear the many sounds going on around you. However, these *sensory* impressions may or may not register in conscious thought.

- You pause in the produce department and consider what fruit is in season at this time of year. You glance at a papaya, a fruit that you have never tried, and notice that it is very expensive. If you then move on, you will probably not recall the papaya in any detail. The impression of the papaya has entered *short-term memory* or consciousness but has not necessarily been stored in long-term memory.

- However, if you pay more attention to the papaya by noting its shape, color, and texture, smelling its fragrance, feeling its ripeness, and even thinking about what it might taste like or how you could prepare it, you will probably transfer the image and knowledge of that fruit into *long-term memory*. This information will be available for retrieval in the future, for example, when you see a recipe that includes papaya as an ingredient.

Remembering: Encoding and Retrieval

Remembering can be defined as learning and storing information so that it can be retrieved at some future time. Thus, *successful* remembering consists of:

1. getting information solidly into long-term memory (encoding) and
2. retrieving information when it is needed.

Note to the Teacher *(Remembering: Encoding and Retrieval)*

After teaching the three stages of memory, the next step is to discuss in more detail how information gets into long-term memory and is recalled at a later time. We have had some concerns over using too many technical terms, but we have decided that older adults deserve to know the terms that are used by researchers today. It is almost impossible to discuss remembering without defining the following terms: encoding, retrieval, attention, association, recall, recognition, and cue. You will find definitions of these terms in *Improving Your Memory,* p. 4–9, 13, and may want to encourage your students to use these terms correctly throughout the course as they work on improving memory.

Let's discuss what is involved in these two aspects of the process of memory.

Encoding

Researchers use the term *encoding* to describe the process of getting information into long-term memory. Encoding may consist of a number of mental tasks, such as paying attention to something, reasoning it through, associating it with something already known, analyzing it, and elaborating on the details. Often these tasks are performed automatically without any conscious effort on our part. These tasks give deeper meaning to the information and strengthen our chances of remembering it. Perhaps the easiest way to understand encoding is to look at the way it works in everyday life.

EXAMPLES

- Mrs. Yang is a confirmed people-watcher. She loves to sit on a park bench and observe life around her. On any given day, she is aware that there are many people in the park walking their dogs. One day a puppy came up and licked her leg. She petted him, felt his soft fur, and enjoyed his exuberance. She asked the owner the puppy's name and breed. She watched as the puppy explored the riverside area. Several days later when she read her grandson a story about a puppy, she recalled the event and described the puppy in the park to him. She was surprised that she remembered the puppy's name and breed so clearly. Although she had no recollection of the many other dogs she saw that day, the information about the puppy had been well encoded because she had been interested, had paid attention, and had elaborated on the details of the interaction.

- On another day in the park, Mrs. Yang sat next to a friendly woman about her age. After sharing a warm conversation, her new friend introduced herself as Mrs. Meadors. Mrs. Yang thought to herself, "I wish I could remember her name as well as I remember the name of the cute puppy I met." Instead of assuming that she couldn't do it, she decided to give it some thought and see if she

---

Additional Example *(Remembering: Encoding and Retrieval)*

Mr. and Mrs. Rundle took a trip to northern Michigan in 1987. During their week's vacation, they visited several villages and beaches along the shore of Lake Michigan. The weather was mostly cold and rainy, with a few episodes of welcome sunshine. On the most beautiful afternoon of the vacation, they took a long walk along a deserted stretch of beach near Harbor Bay. They spent several hours soaking up the sunshine and looking for driftwood and seashells. They noticed that the rocky shoreline included multicolored pebbles and boulders of all sizes worn perfectly smooth by the movement of the waves. They were amazed by the variety and number, for this area was different from the other beaches they had explored. They wondered what natural phenomenon had gifted this area with such beautiful stones. They collected some small stones to take home as souvenirs. They felt especially close to each other and to nature and went to their motel feeling tired and content. Whenever they talk about their trip to northern Michigan in 1987, they recall that day on that beach with great clarity. These memories are particularly strong because they were encoded well and had both intellectual and emotional meaning.

could figure out a way to remember it. When she discovered that Mrs. Meadors grew up on a farm, she thought, "I can picture her in a meadow, which sounds like Meadors." In this example, Mrs. Yang intentionally encoded the information by paying attention to it, analyzing it, and associating it with something already known.

Two tasks of encoding—attention and association—deserve some additional emphasis.

Attention. The first step in the process of encoding information into long-term memory is paying attention. Paying attention is one of the tasks of short-term memory. At any given moment, there are many pieces of information competing for the attention of your short-term memory. It may take some conscious effort on your part to focus your attention on what you need to remember. Keep in mind that the amount of material you can hold in your short-term memory is very limited. You need to zero in on what is important.

EXAMPLES

- A friend tells you to meet her for lunch at 12:00, and you make a note of the date and time in your appointment book. You mistakenly arrive at the restaurant at 12:30 because you didn't pay particular attention when the time was discussed, and you wrote it down incorrectly. Next time, resolve to focus your attention on the details of time and place, and be sure you write them down correctly.

- You were given directions to a new dentist's office and had no trouble finding it the first time. For a second visit, you assume that you will remember where to go. As you approach the area, you realize that you don't know which high-rise building his office is in. What has happened is that you didn't pay enough attention to the

Note to the Teacher *(Attention)*

Because there are often many stimuli competing for our attention, we sometimes find that we have paid attention to the wrong thing and have missed what we really want to remember. For example, you're attending a workshop on memory improvement. All of a sudden you notice that you've been staring at a woman's unusual clothing instead of paying attention to the lecture. A week later you still recall the purple sequined sweater worn with red sweatpants, and have no recollection of how depression affects memory. Focusing attention on what you really want to remember is a first step in improving memory. Encourage your students to be aware of whether inattention may be affecting their abilities to remember.

"The true art of memory is the art of attention."
—Samuel Johnson

"Memory is a crazy woman that hoards colored rags and throws away food."
—Austin O'Malley

Additional Example *(Attention)*

You talked to a friend on the phone and made plans to meet at her home one evening to watch a video together. You offered to pick up the video, and she suggested *Dances with Wolves*. When you got to the video store, you realized that you had no recollection of the name of the movie. What happened is that you didn't pay adequate attention to the title and assumed you would recall it when you needed to. More focused attention would have solved this problem.

location and the appearance of the building. In the future, note some landmarks and descriptive features that will differentiate one building from the next.

In both of these examples the subjects believed that they were paying enough attention to encode the information sufficiently, but clearly they weren't. Everyone has had this experience many times. We give superficial attention to a piece of information and then are frustrated when we can't remember it exactly. One of the simplest ways to improve your memory is to realize the importance of focusing your attention on what you really want to remember. In the future, when you forget, ask yourself if the problem was inadequate attention.

Association. Another aspect of encoding that deserves some explanation is association. Whether we are aware of it or not, new information is encoded by connecting it with other well-known and relevant information that already exists in long-term memory. This process is called association. The easiest way to understand the concept of association is to look at how it happens effortlessly in daily life.

EXAMPLES

• If you meet a new person, your memory of him may be encoded by making a number of different associations. You note what he looks like; where you met him; where he lives; what kind of work he does; and any friends you have in common. Thus an association could be made with these different classifications: curly haired people; the theater where you met him; other people who live in his neighborhood; the medical profession; or the woman who introduced him to you. In the future, thinking of any of these categories could trigger a recollection of your new acquaintance. When you see another curly haired person, or a doctor, or go to the theater, the experience may serve as a cue, and you may think of your new acquaintance.

Note to the Teacher *(Association)*

Association can be a slightly difficult concept to teach. Everyone makes associations, but they may not recognize that they can consciously create associations as a technique for remembering. While teaching this course, you will find it is helpful to use association in your own life. Accept the challenge of creating new associations that can be used as examples in your memory course. The more examples you can give, the clearer this concept will become. Students should also be encouraged to share examples of their successful use of association with class members.

Additional Examples *(Association)*

Suppose you are hearing a lecture on foot care for people with diabetes. Your chances of encoding this new information are greatly increased if you know someone who has diabetes and has had foot ulcers, and if you know something about the complications of diabetes. These associations will make the new information more meaningful and easier to remember. Without any such associations, information about foot care is less likely to be stored in your long-term memory. Thus information about which you have little related knowledge is difficult to recall at a later time. The more associations you are able to make, the more likely you are to remember the information.

Your grandson is fascinated by the children's TV show "Sesame Street." You recently bought a book for him about many of the Sesame Street characters. When he points to each character, asking for the name, you want to be able to answer. You find it difficult to differentiate between Bert and Ernie, two characters who are always seen together. In looking for ways to associate the names with the characters, you notice that Bert has a much bigger head than Ernie. You think, "Bert—big! Both words begin with *B*. That's how I'll remember."

- Suppose your granddaughter has recently been chosen to be on the high-school field-hockey team. You don't know anything about how the game is played or the equipment that's used. However, you do know something about football. When your granddaughter explains the game and equipment to you, you automatically associate the new information about field size, scoring, timekeeping, and protective equipment with what you already know about football. Without any such associations, information about field hockey would be difficult to encode. The next time you watch football on TV, you may think of your conversation with your granddaughter and remember that she has a field-hockey game coming up.

Much association of new information is done unconsciously, but you can make a conscious effort to associate something you want to remember with something you already know. The more effort you put into creating these associations and the greater the number of cross-references available, the more likely you are to recall at will. In Chapter 4, on memory improvement techniques, we will discuss how you can use association to help you remember.

Retrieval

Retrieval is the process of getting information from long-term memory into the conscious state of short-term memory. Most memory complaints center on the inability to bring to mind information on demand. In actuality, however, our ability to find a piece of information in our vast storehouse of memories and bring it to awareness is truly amazing and happens easily most of the time.

There are two ways by which information you have processed and stored in long-term memory is retrieved.

"The more other facts a fact is associated with in the mind, the better possession of it our memory retains. Each of its associations becomes a hook to which it hangs, a means to fish it up by when sunk beneath the surface. Together, they form a network of attachments by which it is woven into the entire tissue of our thought. The 'secret of good memory' is thus the secret of forming diverse and multiple associations with every fact we care to retain."
—William James

Supplementary Material *(Retrieval)*

We all have learned that one way to recall something we have forgotten is to go back to the place where we first thought of it. For example, if I leave the kitchen to do something in my bedroom and can't remember what I planned to do by the time I get there, I may need to return to the kitchen to retrieve the original thought. The thought is more easily recalled if you reinstate the external environment.

Likewise, events or thoughts are more easily recalled when a person's internal environment is similar to the one in which the original thought or event occurred. This is called *state-dependent memory*. For example, when you are in a happy state, you are more likely to recall happy events of the past. In a depressed or anxious state, past events that are depressing or anxiety-producing tend to crowd to the surface.

Recall: a self-initiated search of long-term memory for information

Recognition: perceiving information that is presented to you as something or someone you already know

In most cases recognition is easier than recall. When you say "I can't remember," you usually mean "I can't recall." Even though you cannot recall the name of your representative in Congress, you may easily recognize it when you see it. It may be hard to recall the name of a particular TV show, but you recognize it easily when you see it in the *TV Guide.*

Recall of information is often triggered by a cue. A cue is an event, thought, picture, word, sound, or so forth that triggers the retrieval of information from long-term memory. For example, you may be able to recall the last name of your congressman when prompted with his first name. This triggering information, his first name, is a cue.

People often say, "I can't remember names, but I never forget a face." The reason we remember faces easily is that they present themselves for *recognition.* Remembering names, on the other hand, involves *recall* of information from long-term memory, for which the face is only a cue. When we are searching for a name or other piece of information, we can think of related facts, which may serve as cues, and will often trigger the desired piece of information. For example, if you are having trouble recalling what course you took in summer school, you might think about where it was held, who was in the class with you, and the subjects you have taken in the past.

Exercise for In-Class Use *(Retrieval)*

This is another exercise to demonstrate recall versus recognition. Read the questions to the class and ask them to write down the answers. Then ask the questions again, giving the multiple choice answers. Discuss whether participants found it easier to recognize or to recall the answers.

1. What is the capital city of Illinois?
   Chicago
   Peoria
   Springfield
   Champaign

2. Who was the male star of the movie *Casablanca?*
   Humphrey Bogart
   Gary Cooper
   Clark Gable
   Jimmy Cagney

3. Who wrote the book *Little Women?*
   Emily Brontë
   Louisa May Alcott
   Loretta Aldrich
   Jane Austen

4. What is the name of the labor leader who mysteriously disappeared from Detroit in 1975?
   Roy Cohn
   Abbie Hoffman
   Jimmy Hoffa
   Richard Daley

EXERCISE: RECALL

In order to answer the following questions you are required to recall *the information from long-term memory. If you find this task difficult, try to see if you can* recognize *the correct answers to the questions as they are asked again on p. 13.*

1. What is the name of the hometown of the comic strip character Lil' Abner?

_____

2. Who played Dorothy in the movie *The Wizard of Oz?*

_____

3. What is the name of the island in the Pacific Ocean which is famous for a photograph taken of U.S. Marines raising the American flag after a fierce battle with the Japanese?

_____

4. Who was vice-president of the United States in Richard Nixon's first administration?

_____

See p. 95 for answers.

Exercise for In-Class Use *(Retrieval)*

The following exercise is both instructional and fun. It demonstrates one of the ways that information is stored and how easily information can be triggered with a good cue. Below you will find a column listing categories of words followed by a column of corresponding letters. Make enlarged copies of Set 1 and Set 2 and give them to participants. Ask them to write down a word that fits each category beginning with the corresponding letter; for example, name a fruit beginning with the letter *P.* This exercise should be completed within ninety seconds.

Set 1

Fruit	P	Boy's name	H
Animal	D	Girl's name	M
Metal	I	Vegetable	P
Bird	B	Weapon	S
Country	F	Flower	P

After everyone has worked on Set 1, you might ask them how easy or difficult it was to do this exercise. We have found that most people can complete Set 1 fairly easily. Ask participants to call out their answers as you read the list of categories.

Next, ask participants to work on Set 2 with the following change in instructions: name a word that fits the category ending with the corresponding letter, for example, name a fruit *ending* with the letter *H.* You may want to give people a little longer to complete Set 2, because it is more difficult. It is not important that people have an answer for each category.

Set 2

Fruit	H	Boy's name	D
Animal	W	Girl's name	N
Metal	R	Vegetable	T
Bird	N	Weapon	W
Country	Y	Flower	T

Ask participants to call out answers as you read the list of categories. Most people will find this task much more difficult and will be unable to come up

Forgetting

It is important to recognize that no one can remember everything. An essential part of the memory process is making decisions about what information is valuable and worth the effort it takes to encode it. Is it really critical to spend energy in encoding the name of a woman who occasionally teaches your exercise class when she is only an infrequent substitute? It might be better to choose to learn the names of your grandson's new wife and her parents.

Most people feel very frustrated and even embarrassed when they have to say, "I've forgotten." However, before you blame a faulty memory, it's important to understand that there are some good reasons for not remembering.

1. *Some information never gets into the memory bank.* It only gets as far as sensory memory or short-term memory. Why? You didn't pay attention to it. You didn't really hear it. You didn't understand it. You didn't care enough to remember it. You got distracted by something else. You didn't need to remember it.

2. *Memories that do enter the memory bank may be overladen with subsequent similar information that makes the original memory irretrievable.* People often describe their inadequacies in memory by saying, "I can't even remember what I ate for breakfast yesterday." If you eat similar types of breakfast food day after day, you may forget what you ate on any particular morning, while the memory of the one time you ate octopus remains firm.

3. *Information for which you have few associations and little background knowledge is harder to remember.* For example, if you are just a beginner at the game of bridge, you will find it hard to remember any particular hand dealt during an evening of play, but a bridge expert can accurately recall all of the cards in a particularly meaningful hand.

4. *Some information may only be remembered when the proper cues are available, and those cues are not part of everyday life.* For example, you may think you've forgotten many of your eighth-grade classmates until you find an old photo or go to a class reunion.

5. *It is believed that some memories fade away.* They are not readily

with an answer for each category. At the end of this exercise, you can discuss the fact that first letters are very good cues for most people, while last letters give very little information that will cue a desired word.

(Exercise adapted with permission from Alan Baddeley, *Your Memory: A User's Guide* [New York: Macmillan, 1982].)

"The art of being wise is the art of knowing what to overlook."
—William James

Supplementary Material *(Forgetting)*

Many people assume that their own memories are a true picture of what really happened and are upset or confused by the conflicting recollections of others. In the student text, we discuss how memories change over time, but there are also individual differences that affect encoding of information. Our background, previous knowledge, training, stance on life, age, gender, and prejudices—all have an impact on the way we interpret events and commit them to memory. When two people remember things differently, they may argue over who is "forgetting." In reality, the difference in recollection may be due to the differing views and experiences of the participants. For example, in intergenerational conflict, the middle-aged child may assume that his elderly parent has forgotten what "really happened," when the differences in memory are due to their differing perspectives.

available for all time. For example, if you studied a foreign language in high school, you may recall or recognize many of the vocabulary words you learned. However, there undoubtedly are many other words you have no recollection of and no longer recognize.

6. *Memories change over time.* A common misconception is that information stored in long-term memory remains stable. If an event is recounted from time to time over a number of years, we are more likely to retain a memory of it; however, the content of the memory is also likely to be changed. As we reflect upon it, we unconsciously reconstruct it based on what has happened to us in the interim. This explains why participants in the same event often have very different recollections of it after time has passed.

Review of Terms

Let's review some of the terms used to describe the memory process.

Sensory: referring to the five senses through which all information enters the brain

Short-term memory: equated with conscious thought, it holds the very small amount of information you can pay attention to at a given moment

Long-term memory: the accumulation of information that is not present in conscious thought but is stored for potential recollection

Encoding: learning and storing information

Retrieval: bringing information from long-term memory to conscious thought

Association: the connection between new information and what you already know

Recall: a self-initiated search of long-term memory for information

Recognition: perceiving information that is presented to you as something or someone you already know

Cue: the event, thought, picture, word, sound, and so on that triggers the retrieval of information from long-term memory

Supplementary Material *(Forgetting)*

Students often ask about the role of repression in forgetting. This concept originated with Freud, who believed that forgetting is often due to repression of memories of painful or anxiety-producing events. While memory experts recognize that there are many other reasons for forgetting, there are times when people do repress uncomfortable or painful memories. Research suggests that for most people incidents associated with pain and anxiety will be forgotten more readily than those associated with pleasure. Sometimes, however, people have great difficulty forgetting unpleasant events because of obsessional thinking about the event.

EXERCISE: RECOGNITION

In order to answer the following questions you are required to
recognize *the correct answers.*

1. What is the name of the hometown of the comic strip
   character Lil' Abner?
   > Spring Hill
   > Dogpatch
   > Daisyville

2. Who played Dorothy in the movie *The Wizard of Oz?*
   > Doris Day
   > Judy Holliday
   > Judy Garland

3. What is the name of the island in the Pacific Ocean which is
   famous for a photograph taken of U.S. Marines raising the
   American flag after a fierce battle with the Japanese?
   > Oahu
   > Iwo Jima
   > Guam

4. Who was vice-president of the United States in Richard
   Nixon's first administration?
   > John Agnes
   > Spiro Agnew
   > Gerald Ford

See p. 95 for answers.

EXERCISE: UNDERSTANDING THE MEMORY PROCESS

Complete the blanks in this scenario to test your understanding of the memory process. Use the words listed below.

cue

sensory memory

association

encoding

long-term memory

short-term memory

retrieval

When you go to the library and notice that there are a lot of colorful books on the "new books" shelf, you are using

_____ .

You read through the titles and think about whether they interest you. These conscious thoughts occur in

_____ .

Then you notice a book by a favorite author, James Michener. You take down the book, notice how long it is, read the dust jacket, and decide that you don't have time to read it this month. This process is called

_____ .

The information about the book leaves your conscious thought and goes into

_____ ,

where it may be available for

_____

at another time. When you get home, you notice another of Michener's books in your den. This favorite book serves as a

_____

and reminds you of the book in the library. The connection between the library book and your book is called

_____ .

See p. 95 for answers.

EXERCISE: HOW MEMORY WORKS

True/False. Circle the answer.

T   F   1. Short-term memory refers to something that happened within the last two days.

T   F   2. All information in conscious thought becomes part of your long-term memory.

T   F   3. Sensory impressions may not register in conscious thought.

T   F   4. Associations are made both consciously and unconsciously.

T   F   5. One piece of new information can be associated with many different facts in your long-term memory.

T   F   6. When you are presented with a name that you perceive as something you know, this form of retrieval is called recognition.

T   F   7. Once information is encoded in long-term memory, it doesn't change.

See p. 96 for answers.

2 How Memory Changes as People Age

There are many myths about the inevitability of "senility" as people age, but the truth is that the large majority of older people will not face severe memory loss. Sensory memory exhibits little change as people grow older. Older adults usually can register information through their senses in the same way they did when they were younger. The short-term memory capacity is much the same in older and younger people. Thus, an older person experiences little change in her ability to look up an address in her club directory and address an envelope, a task that requires only sensory and short-term memory.

The memory difficulties that most older people describe involve:

Encoding: getting information solidly into long-term memory;
   "I can't remember what I read as well as I used to."

Recall: retrieving information on demand;
   "I know the name of my medicine, but I can't think of it now."

On the other hand, most older people do not describe problems with recognition.

   "I know it when I see it," or "I know it when I hear it."

Although there is considerable variability among all people in terms of memory, many older people can expect changes in the following areas:

Chapter 2: HOW MEMORY CHANGES AS PEOPLE AGE

Extensive research has been carried out to determine the ways that memory changes with age. Most current studies ask very precise and distinct research questions that aim to collect data about specific aspects of memory, such as spatial memory, memory for faces, and memory for discourse. The sum of this research has enabled memory experts to make some general statements about the memory changes that occur with age. We have chosen to focus on the memory changes that seem most relevant to the older adults we have worked with over the last ten years.

Divided attention: It becomes more difficult to pay attention to more than one thing at a time.

Learning new information: It takes greater effort to learn something new.

Retrieval: It is increasingly difficult to access familiar names and vocabulary words on demand.

Recall: It takes longer to recall information from long-term memory.

Accumulation of knowledge: People gain knowledge and wisdom with age.

In this chapter we'll look at each of these five ways that memory changes with age.

It Becomes More Difficult to Pay Attention to More Than One Thing at a Time

As you grow older you may find it harder to attend to two competing activities, thoughts, or conversations. Keep in mind that the amount of information that can be held in short-term memory is very limited, so what you are thinking of can even be displaced by your own new thought. Also, distractions such as a radio playing, someone talking, or a doorbell ringing may disrupt your concentration more now than they used to.

── EXAMPLES ──

• You are in the middle of a discussion at a party when you hear your name mentioned in a nearby conversation. This momentary distraction makes you lose track of what you are saying. You may feel embarrassed and blame your failing memory, but what has actually occurred is that one thought has displaced another in your short-term memory. This is a common experience, and you can simply say," Where was I? I lost my train of thought."

Note to the Teacher *(It Becomes More Difficult to Pay Attention)*

As you teach about difficulty in paying attention to more than one thing at a time, you may need to review the concept of short-term memory. Remind students that short-term memory refers to the very small amount of information that you can hold in your mind, or pay attention to, at one time and that this information can be easily displaced by a new thought. Give several examples of how inadequate attention or distractions can lead to forgetting.

- You have several questions you need to ask your doctor when you see him. When he enters the exam room, you have them well in mind. Then he starts asking you questions about your health. You find that you no longer remember *your* questions. Remembering what you intend to ask your doctor at the same time that you are answering his questions involves a division of attention. If you go to your doctor with a written list of your questions, you will not have to rely on your memory.

EXERCISE: DIVIDED ATTENTION

Can you add this column of figures while you continually repeat the names of the months of the year?

$$
\begin{array}{r}
4 \\
8 \\
5 \\
7 \\
\underline{9} \\
\end{array}
$$

This exercise demonstrates how difficult it is to pay attention to two fairly simple tasks at one time.

 ASSIGNMENT ━━━━━━━━━━━━━━━━

During the next few days, notice if your attention is divided while you are trying to read the evening paper or listen to the news. Perhaps the phone rings or you jump up to stir the soup. Maybe your spouse asks you a question. Think about whether these distractions affect your ability to remember what you are reading or listening to. Is it a problem with your memory or are you trying to attend to too many things at once?

Additional Examples *(It Becomes More Difficult to Pay Attention)*

You are in the middle of baking bread when the thought of a old friend comes into your mind. You daydream for a moment about your last visit together. When you return to your baking, you realize that you're not sure how many cups of flour you have added.

You are listening to the baseball game on the radio, eager to catch the score at the end of the inning. At the same time, you are sorting through the mail. It seems perfectly reasonable to do these two things at once, but you suddenly realize the inning is over and you missed hearing the score. In this case, focus your attention on the game until the score is announced, then finish sorting through the mail.

It Takes Greater Effort to Learn Something New

Although we know that some information enters long-term memory without effort or awareness, much new learning takes conscious effort and an intent to learn. Too many people believe the myth that "you can't teach an old dog new tricks," but, unless there is impairment of the brain, people can continue to learn and remember throughout life. There are many strategies, some of which will be discussed later in this book, for organizing new information and giving it meaning in order to solidly store it in long-term memory. However, researchers have found that older adults may not spontaneously use the most effective strategies for memory performance. Information that you could learn with little effort in the past may now require greater effort in order to remember. After you decide that it is important for you to remember some new information, you must focus your attention on the task and find some means of encoding the information. As you recall from chapter 1, encoding may include paying attention to something, reasoning it through, analyzing it, associating it with something already known, and elaborating on the details.

EXAMPLE

• Your city council has just enacted new regulations regarding collection of recycled plastic. They will now accept certain plastic containers at curbside, while others are unacceptable. You regularly use, and would like to recycle, detergent, bleach, milk, cottage cheese, and yogurt containers. Because you keep forgetting which items are acceptable, you end up throwing them all in the trash. You decide that you want to easily remember which items to recycle without looking up the regulations each time or asking your neighbor. The first step in learning this new information is giving your undivided attention to reading the information leaflet from the recycling center. You focus on the portion that describes what to do with plastics. The next step is thinking about how you can

Note to the Teacher *(It Takes Greater Effort)*

When teaching about using greater effort to learn new information, it's important to stress that the concept of "greater effort" is both individual and undefined. Even the concept of "normal effort" varies greatly from individual to individual, as does the individual's expectations for mastery. In each new learning situation, a person must determine

• what information is important to remember
• what level of learning constitutes mastery
• how much effort is actually required to achieve his own goals
• whether the accomplishment is worth the effort required

One way to help people see individual differences might be to assign a short article to be read in class. Ask students to answer the above questions for themselves after reading the headlines only. Helen may find the topic irrelevant and not worth any effort; Frank may state that he would only like to find out the conclusions drawn by the author; Judith may want to be able to quote statistics to persuade her friends of her viewpoint; Kenneth may think the topic is interesting but state that he has never enjoyed reading and doesn't want to expend any effort. You might ask those students who are interested in the article to read through it quickly and find out if their expectations for learning are met. If not, they need to assess how much effort is required to meet their goals.

remember which of your commonly collected plastic items can go in the recycling bin. You note that the milk, bleach, and detergent containers are acceptable, whereas the cottage cheese and yogurt containers are not. After analyzing the situation, you realize that the three acceptable plastic items all contain liquids, whereas the others contain solids. Grouping these containers into other classifications, such as color, size, or shape, might also produce a solution to your problem. You could easily have said, "It's too complicated for me. I can't remember all these distinctions." Instead you decided that it was important to learn and found a means of encoding the information.

EXERCISE: LEARNING NEW INFORMATION

Here is some new information for you to learn and remember. Give it your undivided attention and see how much effort it requires for you to answer the questions that follow the reading. Even though the particular subject may not interest you, the challenge is to find a way to remember the material even if it takes greater effort than you thought it would.

Social Network Size Matters, Jobs Study Shows

For older people seeking work, a University of Southern California research team suggests that a key factor in landing a job is not only who you know, but how many. The more relatives and friends older job-seekers had, the study found, the more likely they were to find work.

The researchers, led by assistant professor of social work Michal Mor-Barak, Ph.D., interviewed 146 Los Angeles–area men and women 55 and older who a year earlier had signed up at

---

Additional Example *(It Takes Greater Effort)*

Mrs. Campbell has two friends named Gail, one from her bridge club and the other from her neighborhood. She knows that one of them spells her name Gayle, but she can never remember which one. The spelling of the names is only important when she sends her yearly holiday cards. Since she knows them very well, she would be embarrassed if she misspelled their names. She decides that she wants to be spared this yearly quandary. She says to herself, "There must be a way to remember who is who." She calls a friend who says that Gail from the bridge club spells her name Gayle. She analyzes the spelling of the names and thinks about each person's characteristics. She realizes that GaYle is younger than Gail. "*Y* stands for younger!" she exclaims. She paid attention to the spelling of the names; she figured out a way to create an association between the spelling and the women; and she repeated the association aloud. All of these efforts resulted in deeply encoding the spelling of the names.

various public-service agencies for help in finding work. All had retired, lost their jobs, or were trying to re-enter the workforce for reasons ranging from financial need to boredom. The study found that 64 percent got jobs.

Besides social network size, other factors predicting success at finding work were high motivation and a low number of major life changes such as divorce, marriage, death of a family member or close friend.

Half of those surveyed were white, half roughly equal numbers of Hispanics, blacks and Asians. They were better educated than the general population: 40 percent had attended college: 24 percent had degrees, and some of those had advanced degrees.

The study concluded that it's important for older job-seekers to get connected. One route is via a support group, where they can learn from others' experiences and discuss ways to deal with obstacles such as age discrimination.

(Reprinted with permission from *Modern Maturity*. Copyright 1992, American Association of Retired Persons.)

1. What are the most important factors in finding a job?

2. Name another key factor in finding work.

3. Did more than half of the 146 people surveyed find jobs?

4. What is one conclusion of the study?

See p. 96 for answers.

It Is Increasingly Difficult to Access Familiar Names and Vocabulary Words on Demand

Everyone knows the experience of being halted in mid-sentence when the desired word or name does not immediately spring to mind. The feeling of the word being on the tip of your tongue occurs more frequently as you age. The frustration of this experience can make you feel anxious, and this anxiety further blocks the recall process.

EXAMPLES

- You begin to tell a friend about the movie you saw last night and you're astonished and embarrassed to discover that the title has escaped you. The more irritated you become, the less likely you are to be able to come up with the name. Instead of giving yourself time and cues to retrieve the name of the movie from long-term memory, you find your attention focused on the frustration of forgetting. If you relax and are patient, the information will often come to you.

- You start to tell a friend about the new bird feeder that you put up. "I saw a beautiful cardinal at the bird feeder on my . . ." At that moment the word "porch" escapes you, and you get flustered and say "the outside of my living room." This is a common occurrence that happens to everyone but is experienced more frequently as you grow older.

The next time you find yourself searching for a needed name or word, try to relax, take a deep breath, and see if you can access the information by thinking of related items. If you are still unable to retrieve that needed word, don't fret. It will undoubtedly come to you unbidden while you are thinking of something else.

Note to the Teacher *(It Is Increasingly Difficult to Access Familiar Names and Words)*

Everyone has had the experience of trying to greet or introduce a familiar person and being unable to come up with the name on demand. In our memory course, we encourage people to reintroduce themselves by name when they meet an acquaintance, rather than waiting as the person struggles or, even worse, testing him by asking, "Do you remember me?" Class discussion makes it evident that the problem of accessing familiar names is a common occurrence, and participants are reassured and relieved by the shared experience.

Additional Examples *(It Is Increasingly Difficult to Access Familiar Names and Words)*

You are discussing your college-age grandchildren with your brother. He asks what your grandson Robert is studying. You know what the subject matter is, and you know it starts with *P*. You are embarrassed that you can't come up with "philosophy" and can only think of the word "psychology." This is a fairly common phenomenon. Sometimes a similar word interferes with your ability to find the word you want.

You want to send a birthday card to your niece, who recently married her childhood sweetheart. All of a sudden you can't come up with her married name. You begin to search your memory bank for information about her husband. You think about when you first met him; what he looks like; what kind of work he does; what you know about his family. You recall that his grandfather used to own a family dairy, then it springs to mind—Hamilton's Dairy. Your niece's new name is Yvonne Hamilton. You have used a number of cues to trigger the retrieval of the information you needed from long-term memory.

Note to the Teacher *(It Is Increasingly Difficult to Access Familiar Names and Words)*

Students sometimes ask whether it is harder to retrieve names and words when you are older because you have too much information in the memory bank. You can reassure your students that there is no limit to the amount of

It Takes Longer to Recall Information from Long-Term Memory

Studies have shown that older adults take more time to recall needed information from long-term memory than younger people. When older adults are given increased time to complete a test, their performances are greatly improved. In untimed tests of recall, older adults perform comparably to younger ones. Keep this in mind when you are impatient with yourself because you don't recall something immediately. Give yourself a little additional time and see if you can come up with the desired information.

EXAMPLE

- Mrs. Chen was given a video recorder for her birthday. She read the instruction manual and learned to follow the steps for its use. She taped her favorite shows regularly for several weeks and felt confident in her ability to record the programs she wanted. When she returned from a two-week trip to visit her son in New Jersey, she began to tape a show on cooking. She was frustrated to discover that she was unable to either recall the steps or find the instruction manual. She decided to give it one more try. As she held the remote control in her hand and tried to think back to her prevacation routine, the steps came back to her bit by bit. She thought to herself, "I'm so glad I didn't give up because I couldn't remember right away."

Expertise and familiarity often more than compensate in a specific area for the slowing down of recall. For example, a seventy-year-old crossword-puzzle buff, who spends some time every day in this endeavor, may be able to recall words commonly needed in crossword puzzles as quickly as or more quickly than most younger people.

information that can be stored in long-term memory. However, the volume of information stored may make access more difficult. For example, in order to come up with a particular name, a nine-year-old girl may only need to sort through a circle of acquaintances that includes her family members, classmates, scout troop, and neighbors. On the other hand, an older adult who has stored thousands of names throughout a lifetime may have more difficulty searching for one particular name.

Additional Example *(It Takes Longer to Recall Information from Long-Term Memory)*

Mrs. Whitehouse was talking to her daughter-in-law Jane on the telephone. Jane asked, "What did you do last night?" Mrs. Whitehouse hesitated, then responded, "Well, I guess, . . . nothing." Several seconds later, she exclaimed, "Oh, yeah, we went to see a movie. I just couldn't think of it for a minute." This information was clearly not forgotten; it just took Mrs. Whitehouse a little longer to retrieve it from long-term memory.

People Gain Knowledge and Wisdom with Age

World knowledge, which is defined as a pool of information acquired over a lifetime from both educational and everyday experiences, accumulates with age. In tests that measure knowledge and vocabulary, older adults do as well as or better than younger people. The experiences of a long and rich life can produce a wisdom that young people can only hope to obtain. Memory and experience are the basis of wisdom. Although it takes greater effort to learn something new, older adults have the wisdom to determine what new information is important to them.

EXERCISE: HOW MEMORY CHANGES

True/False. Circle the answer.

T   F   1. There is no escaping "senility" as you grow older.

T   F   2. If you have always been able to do several things at once, age won't affect this ability.

T   F   3. Sensory and short-term memory exhibit little change as people grow older.

T   F   4. Older adults take longer to recall information from long-term memory.

T   F   5. Older adults spontaneously use memory strategies more often than younger adults.

T   F   6. One way to access well-known information when you can't recall it is to provide yourself with cues by thinking of related items.

See p. 96 for answers.

---

3 Factors Affecting Memory for People of All Ages

It is known that certain factors can affect the memory process for people of all ages. However, the impact of these factors is likely to be greater as you age, because older people often experience more of these negative influences at one time. We have identified the following factors that commonly affect memory:

- problems with attention
- negative expectations
- stress
- anxiety
- depression
- loss and grief
- inactivity
- lack of organization in daily life
- fatigue
- some physical illnesses
- some medications
- vision and hearing problems
- alcohol
- poor nutrition

As you read through this section, think about which of these factors might be affecting your memory. Awareness of possible causes of memory problems can lead to solutions.

This section of the memory course is useful in helping people to consider the impact of various factors on memory. In addition, it is a good opportunity to increase knowledge about topics that may affect the general well-being of older adults. For example, participants may not choose to come to a lecture on depression, but in the discussion of how depression can affect memory, they will gain some information that may be vital to themselves or others they know. If time allows, you may want to include presentations by professionals in your community who can address these factors in greater depth, such as a pharmacist, a nutritionist, a psychiatrist, a counselor of older adults, or an expert in stress management.

Problems with Attention

Inadequate Attention

In the discussion of how memory works in Chapter 1, we emphasized the importance of focusing attention on what you want to remember. If you really want to remember something, paying adequate attention is the first step. Here are some examples where inadequate attention affected the encoding of new information.

EXAMPLES

- Connie may be daydreaming when her husband asks her to pick up the dry cleaning. Later, when he asks for his suit, she doesn't even remember the request.

- A new resident of Brad's apartment building, Jane Blair, meets him at the mailboxes and introduces herself. He greets her by name and begins a friendly conversation. When they are joined by another resident a few minutes later, Brad discovers that he has no recollection of Jane's name.

The problem in these two examples is that Connie and Brad have not paid enough attention to encoding the needed information so that they can recall it. Paying adequate attention to details can eliminate some instances of forgetting. Ask yourself, "When is it really important for me to pay attention?" At these times, resolve to focus your awareness on the task or information at hand.

Note to the Teacher *(Problems with Attention)*

The area of attention is a very important one to address in helping people improve their memories. Throughout the course, we stress the concept that you cannot pay attention to everything and must choose to pay attention to what *you* think is important to remember. One participant may feel threatened about constantly misplacing her glasses. Encourage her to pay attention to where she puts them when she removes them. Another participant may consider losing her glasses a minor inconvenience. She may not choose to put any effort toward this task. Help your students to realize that focusing attention in areas of individual importance is a basic and powerful way to alleviate problems with forgetting.

Additional Example *(Inadequate Attention)*

Mr. Gregory's neighbor asks him to feed her cat while she is gone over the weekend. She tells him where the cat food is kept, how much and how often to feed her, and where she hides the spare key. When Mr. Gregory goes to feed that cat, he is horrified to discover that he does not recall where the key is hidden. Because he is unfamiliar with cats, he paid close attention to the instructions regarding feeding, but he assumed that he would remember where the key was hidden and paid little attention to that detail.

Distractions

As you recall from chapter 1, paying attention is one of the tasks of short-term memory. It is important to remember that the amount of information that can be held in your short-term memory is very limited. Any new sound, sight, or thought may distract you and displace what is currently in your short-term memory.

EXAMPLES

- You are certain to have had the experience of going into another room and forgetting what you went for. As you went into the kitchen to get the scissors, perhaps you thought, "I wonder if the mail is here." This new thought replaced the thought of the scissors you needed from the kitchen.

- When you leave your umbrella in the doctor's office, it may be because you are thinking of getting your prescription filled before the drugstore closes.

- You're driving to a movie with a friend. Her conversation draws your attention from noticing exactly where you are, and you forget to get into the left turn lane until it's too late. To avoid this frustrating experience, you might want to ask your passenger to hold her conversation until you get to the movie theater.

These experiences are familiar to people of all ages, but keep in mind that older adults find it more difficult to pay attention to more than one thing at a time. Rather than thinking you can do nothing about these frustrating experiences, try to recognize the limitations of short-term memory and cut out distractions when possible. It is especially important to give your undivided attention to situations that could be potentially dangerous, such as driving, cooking, and taking medications.

Additional Examples *(Distractions)*

Mr. Schwartz stopped at the store after work to pick up something for dinner. As he went through the check-out line, he began thinking of what TV programs he would watch after dinner. When he got home, he noticed that his small bag of groceries was not in his car. He realized that, while thinking of the TV programs, he forgot to pick up the grocery bag from the check-out counter.

Corinne leaves her house to do some errands, intending to mail a letter at the corner mailbox. As she approaches the mailbox, she realizes that she has left an overdue library book at home. She immediately returns home, locates the book, and continues on her way. Later in the day as she passes the post office, she realizes that she never mailed the letter. Returning home to get the book distracted her from the task of mailing the letter.

EXERCISE: DISTRACTIONS

Below are two short articles. Read the first one in a quiet room, and then read the second one with some competition for your attention, such as the TV or radio.

Fabulous Fakery

Chang Dai-chien, with his floor-length robes, 11th century scholar's cap and four wives (at the same time), cut a striking figure wherever he went. He also attracted much interest as one of the foremost Chinese painters of the 20th century and a skilled forger of ancient masterpieces (he called them "honest copies"). Chang completed almost 30,000 works over a 60-year career that ended with his death in 1983 at the age of 84. A number of Chang's forgeries can be found in collections in the British Museum, Metropolitan Museum of Art and museums throughout China. A retrospective of 87 of his works will be on display at the St. Louis Art Museum (314-721-0072) August 28– October 25.

Ironwoman

Agnes Reinhard, 66, has run many races along Lake Michigan. "Afterward I'd always want to jump in the lake," she says. She gets her wish when she competes August 16 in the Danskin Women's Triathlon Series presented by BMW in Milwaukee— except she jumps in the lake first for a .75K swim, then rides a bike for 20K, and finishes with a 5K run. Reinhard, of West Allis, Wisconsin, placed first in her age division (60-plus) in last year's triathlon and hopes to do as well this year. A personal best to beat? "I don't worry about time," she says. "I compete for the fun of it." More than 7,500 women are expected to enter the Danskin series, the world's only all-women triathlon, which travels to six U.S. cities and Germany.

(Reprinted with permission from *Modern Maturity*. Copyright 1992, American Association of Retired Persons.)

Did you notice a difference in your ability to remember the details?

Negative Expectations

Compared to younger people, older adults are more pessimistic about their *ability* to remember. Older people often say, "I just can't remember anything anymore," whereas younger people attribute forgetting to a lack of *effort*. When you expect that you are going to fail at something, that expectation is likely to increase the possibility of failure. Negative expectations about memory are likely to cause older people to

- put less effort into remembering
- avoid tasks that require memory
- feel anxious when their memories are tested in daily life

EXAMPLE

- Mrs. Martin recently attended a volunteer appreciation banquet. Although she recognized many faces, she felt embarrassed and anxious when she could not address people by name. She thought, "I can't remember names anymore!" Since that time Mrs. Martin has avoided attending gatherings when she doesn't know everyone extremely well. Although her son-in-law gave her a book on how to remember names, she is sure that those techniques are not useful for someone of her age. She stated this belief to her neighbor, who said that she's had the same experience of forgetting familiar names and found a solution. She keeps lists of names of people who are likely to attend various group functions. Before she attends a function, she reviews the appropriate list, visualizing each person. Mrs. Martin agrees to give this technique a try. She is surprised to find that, if she puts enough effort into it, she is able to remember many of the names. She now has more positive expectations about her ability to remember and no longer avoids situations where memory is required. (In chapter 4, you will learn more about remembering names.)

When you are faced with a task of memory, do you find yourself saying, "I'll never be able to do this. What's the use of trying?" Some-

Note to the Teacher *(Negative Expectations)*

You may observe negative expectations in students in your course. If a student is not completing homework assignments or participating in class discussion or exercises, ask yourself if his negative expectations might be affecting his effort. Look for ways to give him feelings of success. On the other hand, be aware that another reason for lack of participation may be that a student is experiencing some organic changes in the brain and is unable to keep up with the demands of the course. You can be supportive of this person's needs by including him in class discussion without putting undue pressure on him.

Additional Example *(Negative Expectations)*

Carolyn was asked by her young friend Ann to join a book club that meets monthly to discuss an assigned book. Carolyn said, "I couldn't possibly be in a group like that. I love to read, but I never remember what I read well enough to talk about it. My memory isn't what it used to be." Ann said, "You know what I do? I make a list of the characters as they enter the story and write down a few words about their roles. After each chapter, I jot down a sentence or two about the plot. At the end, I review my notes, and it refreshes my mind." Carolyn is sure that it won't work, but she agrees to try this method because she wants to please Ann. She is thrilled to find that she can confidently discuss the book after using Ann's strategy. She is so pleased that she gave it a try, because her negative expectations would have kept her from this enjoyable new experience.

times we give ourselves negative messages without being aware of it. Be conscious of your self-defeating thoughts about your ability to remember. Substitute this thought: "I'm not sure this will work, but I'll give it a good try."

Stress

When you are feeling stressed, anxious, pressured, or rushed, it is often impossible to:

- pay adequate attention to learning new information
- concentrate on the details you want to recall
- relax long enough to let a memory surface

You are more likely to forget things when you are under major stress—due to factors such as moving, illness, loss, your own retirement or the retirement of your spouse—or even when you are under minor stress caused by experiences such as being late to an appointment, losing your house keys, preparing for company, or seeing your doctor. It is important to realize that you may forget more frequently at times like these and that your memory usually improves as the stress is reduced. When you add worry about forgetting to other stresses, you often increase forgetfulness.

EXAMPLE

- You have been extremely busy all week getting ready for a visit from your son and his family, who live in California. The sink becomes clogged, and the plumber is only available during the time when you are picking up the family from the airport. You arrange to leave a key with a neighbor so that the work can be done. To your horror, you forget to leave the key when you go to the airport. You are stressed, overloaded, and rushing. Thus you forgot to do what you wanted to do most. In a case like this, it's best to do what you need to do before doing anything else. Leave the key the moment you think of it.

Additional Example *(Stress)*

Mrs. Santiago's husband, Juan, recently had a stroke. He's doing fairly well, but Mrs. Santiago is feeling very stressed. When talking to her son, she complains, "I seem to be losing everything. Yesterday I couldn't find my car keys. My glasses are always disappearing. I can't keep track of who has called. One night I called Juan's sister twice because I'd totally forgotten that I'd already talked to her." The stress in Mrs. Santiago's life is affecting her memory. She can't do anything about that stress right now, but it would be helpful if she recognized that her memory will undoubtedly improve when her stress is reduced.

Anxiety

Anxiety is characterized as inner distress accompanied by physical symptoms and vague fears. Many people who are highly anxious are unable to focus on anything outside of themselves. Their minds are so filled with worries that they cannot pay attention to external happenings, and their memory failures affect their daily functioning.

Some symptoms of anxiety are:

- nervousness, worry, or fear
- apprehension or a sense of imminent doom
- panic spells
- difficulty concentrating
- insomnia
- fear of potential physical illnesses
- heart pounding or racing
- upset stomach or diarrhea
- sweating
- dizziness or light-headedness
- restlessness or jumpiness
- irritability

EXAMPLE

- Eva describes herself as someone who has always been a worrier, but it has gotten worse as she has grown older. She worries about her high blood pressure, her unmarried son, her granddaughter's thumb-sucking, and her arthritis, which could affect her ability to take care of her home. She has butterflies in her stomach; she doesn't sleep well; she spends most of the day worrying; and she is unable to remember things very well. When she is in the clinic to get a blood pressure reading, she mentions her anxiety to the nurse, who suggests that she should discuss it with the doctor. Dr. Persky recommends a cognitive therapy group for people who are anxious or depressed, where she might learn new ways of dealing with her anxiety and benefit from the group support. In the group,

Eva recognizes that she has no control over her son's unmarried state and her granddaughter's thumb-sucking. She is able to take them off her worry list. The group helps her consider some options for the future in case she is unable to take care of her home. Eva knows that she will continue to be a worrier; however, when she realized the uselessness of worrying about those things that she cannot control and began to make plans for her future, some of her symptoms of anxiety were alleviated, including her memory problems.

Depression

Everyone feels blue off and on during a lifetime. However, ongoing depression is not normal and can affect memory. Older people are not necessarily more prone to depression than younger people, but the losses and physical illnesses that frequently accompany old age can rob the older person of the hope of a better future. Some symptoms of depression are:

- appetite change (decrease in appetite is most common)
- sleep disturbance
- fatigue
- anxiety, fearfulness, excessive worrying
- feelings of hopelessness, helplessness
- decreased concentration, difficulty with memory
- difficulty making decisions
- restlessness, pacing
- irritability
- feeling that life is not worth living
- feeling that nothing gives you pleasure
- feeling sick or tired all the time
- sad mood
- suicidal thoughts

Additional Example *(Anxiety)*

Mr. Otis has become increasingly anxious since his retirement four months ago. He finds himself feeling restless much of the time; he lies awake for many hours after going to bed; he has trouble sorting through his bills because he can't concentrate. His biggest complaint, however, is that he can't remember anything. He asks his family doctor if there is anything he can take to improve his memory. His doctor suggests that his anxiety might well be affecting his memory and recommends that he see a counselor to treat his anxious response to retirement.

How does depression affect memory?

Motivation: When you are depressed you don't care about remembering your new neighbor's name, the time of your exercise class, or who's running for city council. None of these things seems important.

Concentration: Even if you want to remember how to fill out your Medicare form, depression can make you feel foggy and unable to focus on the task.

Perception: If you are depressed you may view a few instances of forgetting as a sign that you can't remember anything at all.

EXAMPLE

- Mr. McIntyre has experienced bouts of depression for several years. His friends and family noticed that when he was feeling depressed, he forgot appointments, confused the names of his grandchildren, and couldn't remember what happened the day before. The first few times this occurred, his family wondered if he were getting "senile," but, over time, they noticed that when his depression lifted, his memory improved. Thus, Mr. McIntyre and his family recognized that his memory loss was connected to his depression and probably did not indicate progressive deterioration. Rather than accept depression as a normal part of aging, the family encouraged Mr. McIntyre to see his physician for an evaluation. Dr. Smith recommended that the depression be treated by a combination of medication and counseling. He also suggested that, until Mr. McIntyre's depression improved, he should use as many memory aids as possible.

Note to the Teacher *(Depression)*

Many people don't recognize the symptoms of depression or, when they do, think that it's natural for older adults to be depressed. When teaching about how memory can be affected by depression, you have a good opportunity to help people understand depression, recognize its symptoms in themselves or others, and be aware that there are treatments for this very common illness.

Supplementary Material *(Depression)*

The following material is reprinted with permission from the National Institute on Aging's "Age Page," U.S. Department of Health and Human Services, Public Health Service, National Institutes of Health, 1992.

Depression: A Serious but Treatable Illness

Everyone gets the blues now and then. It's part of life. But when there is little joy or pleasure after visiting with friends or after seeing a good movie, there may be a more serious problem. A depressed mood that stays around for a while, without let-up, can change the way a person thinks or feels. Doctors call this "clinical depression."

Being "down in the dumps" over a period of time like this is not a normal part of growing old, but it is a common problem. An older person who feels this way needs medical help. For most people, depression can be treated successfully. "Talk" therapies, drugs, or other methods of treatment can ease the pain of depression. There is no reason to suffer.

There are many reasons why depression in older people is often missed or untreated. As a person ages, the signs of the disease are much more likely to be dismissed as crankiness or moods of "old age." Depression can also be tricky to recognize. Confusion or attention problems caused by depression can sometimes mimic the symptoms of Alzheimer's disease or other disorders of the brain. Mood changes and common symptoms of depression are sometimes the result of side effects of drugs commonly taken by older patients for high blood pressure and heart disease. Depression in late life also frequently occurs with other chronic diseases, making diagnosis difficult and treatment challenging. Depression in older people may not be easy to diagnose, but it should not be ignored because it typically responds to appropriate treatment.

What to Look For

How do you know when help is needed? After all, older people experience more events and problems that might cause anyone to become "depressed"—deaths of loved ones and friends, being unsure of what to do in retirement, or coping with chronic illness. Usually, though, after a normal period of time grieving or feeling troubled, people resume their daily lives. When a person is clinically depressed, his or her ability to function both mentally and physically is affected, and the trouble may last for weeks, months, or even years.

Here is a list of the most common signs of depression. If several of these symptoms last for more than 2 weeks, see a doctor.

- An "empty" feeling, ongoing sadness and anxiety.
- Tiredness, lack of energy.
- Loss of interest or pleasure in ordinary activities, including sex.
- Sleep problems, including very early morning waking.
- Problems with eating and weight (gain or loss).
- A lot of crying.
- Aches and pains that just won't go away.
- Difficulty concentrating, remembering, or making decisions.
- Feelings that the future looks grim; feeling guilty, helpless, or worthless.
- Irritability.
- Thoughts of death or suicide; a suicide attempt.

Families, friends, and health professionals should look carefully for signs of depression in older people. Symptoms vary widely among people and sometimes depression can hide behind a smiling face. For depressed people who live alone, for instance, feelings of despair or loneliness can change briefly when someone stops by to say hello or during a visit to the doctor. The person may get such a boost from the contact with another individual that, for the moment, the depressive symptoms subside.

Don't ignore the warning signs. At its worst, serious depression can lead to suicide. Statistics show that the rate of completed suicides, about 25 percent of those attempted, is higher for older people than that of the general population. Listen carefully when an older friend or relative complains about being depressed or of people not caring. The person may be telling you that he or she needs help.

What Causes Depression?

There is no single cause of depression. For some people, just one event can bring on the illness. Others seem to become depressed for no clear reason. One way that scientists classify depression is to divide it into two forms: primary and secondary. Primary depression occurs in people who have generally been well but who may show symptoms of depression in response to events beyond their control. A death in the family or sudden illness, for example, might bring on depressed feelings. Also, differences in brain chemistry that affect mood can be a cause of primary depression.

Secondary depression is linked to drugs or certain illnesses. Some medications used to treat arthritis, heart problems, high blood pressure, and cancer can produce depression. The effects of these drugs may not always be clear right away. Scientists also think some illnesses themselves can bring about depression. These include Parkinson's disease, stroke, and hormonal disorders.

Genetics, too, can play a role. Studies show that some forms of depression run in families. Children of depressed parents may be at a higher risk of getting the disease themselves.

Treating Depression

Depression is the most treatable of all mental illnesses. About 60 to 80 percent of depressed people can be treated successfully outside a hospital with psychotherapy alone or with special drugs. Medical research has made great progress in recognizing the problem of depression among older people and devising treatments. In fact, this has led to the development of a new medical specialty—geriatric psychiatry—with doctors trained in the diagnosis and relief of depression in late life.

Depending on the case, various kinds of therapies seem to work. Treatments such as psychotherapy and support groups help people deal with major changes in life, such as retirement, moving, or health problems that require new coping skills and social support. Several short-term (12–20 weeks) "talk" therapies have proven useful. One method helps patients recognize and change negative thinking patterns that have led to the depression. Another approach focuses on improving a patient's relationships with people as a way to reduce depression and feelings of despair. A doctor might also suggest that an older patient use community-based programs such as senior centers, volunteer services, or nutrition programs.

Antidepressant drugs can also help. These medications can improve mood, sleep, appetite, and concentration. There are several types of these drugs available, with doctors favoring medications that may have fewer side effects harmful to older people. Drug therapies often take at least 6 to 12 weeks before there are real signs of progress and may need to be continued for 6 months or longer after symptoms disappear.

Despite their benefits, antidepressant drugs need to be used with great care. Many older people take a number of drugs for other problems. A doctor must know about all prescribed and over-the-counter medications being taken and should be aware of all physical problems. This can help avoid unwanted side effects. Also, remember to take the medication in the proper dose and on the right schedule; if not, the drugs may not work.

"Shock" therapy, or electroconvulsive (ECT) therapy, can also help. While its long-term benefits need more study, ECT can work well as a short-term treatment. New techniques assure that ECT is safe and effective when properly used, not like the scary movie version of years ago.

Prevention

In some cases, major depressive illness can be avoided. This is especially true when depression is linked to life events, such as widowhood and retirement, that occur more often with age. For instance, fostering and maintaining relationships with people over the years can help lessen the effects of losing a spouse. Developing interests or hobbies, staying involved in activities that keep the mind and body active, and keeping in touch with family and friends are all ways to keep major depression at bay.

Overall, physical fitness and a balanced diet are important ways to help avoid illnesses that can bring on disability and depression. Also, following the doctor's prescription on the proper use of medicines will reduce the risk of depression as a drug side effect.

Getting Help

The first step to getting help is to overcome negative attitudes that stand in the way. The subject of mental illness still makes many, especially older people, uncomfortable. Some feel that getting help is a sign of weakness. Many older people, their relatives, or friends mistakenly believe that a depressed person can quickly "snap out of it" or that some people are too old to be helped.

Once the decision is made to get medical advice, start with the family doctor. The doctor, whether in private practice, a clinic, or a health maintenance organization, should decide if there are medical or drug-related reasons for the symptoms of depression. After a complete exam, the physician may refer the older patient to a mental health specialist for further study and possible treatment. Be aware that a few doctors may share some of the negative attitudes about aging and depression and may not be interested in the complaints. Insist that your concerns be taken seriously or find a doctor who is willing to help.

If a depressed older person refuses to go along with evaluation and treatment, relatives or friends can be reassuring. Explain how treatment will reduce symptoms and make the person feel better. In some cases, when an older person can't or won't go to the doctor's office, the doctor or mental health specialist can call and arrange a visit to the patient's home. The telephone is not a substitute for the personal contact needed for a complete medical checkup, but it can break the ice.

Don't avoid seeking help because you are afraid of how much treatment might cost. Often, the problem can be solved with weeks—not months or years—of therapy or medications. Also, community mental health centers offer treatment based on a patient's ability to pay.

For More Information

You can find out more about depression and its treatments by contacting the following organizations.

The National Institute of Mental Health's special DEPRESSION Awareness, Recognition, and Treatment (D/ART) Program offers several publications on depression, including "If You're Over 65 and Feeling Depressed . . . Treatment Brings New Hope." Contact D/ART Public Inquiries, National Institute of Mental Health, 5600 Fishers Lane, Room 15C-05, Rockville, MD 20857.

The National Depressive and Manic-Depressive Association has over 200 chapters in the United States and Canada which offer support to people with depression and their families. They sponsor education and research programs and distribute brochures, videotapes, and audio programs. Write to the Association at P.O. Box 1939, Chicago IL 60690; (800) 826-3632.

The National Alliance for the Mentally Ill has a Medical Information Series that provides patients and families with information on several mental illnesses and their treatments, including a publication "Mood Disorders: Depression and Manic Depression." NAMI groups in all states provide emotional support and can help people find appropriate local services. Write or call NAMI at 2101 Wilson Boulevard, Suite 302, Arlington, VA 22201; (800) 950-NAMI (6264).

The National Mental Health Association also publishes information on a variety of mental health issues. It has special information on depression and its treatment, and provides referrals and support. Write or call NMHA, Information Center, 1021 Prince Street, Alexandria, VA 22314-2971; (800) 969-6642.

The National Institute on Aging offers information on a range of health issues that concern older people. Write to the NIA Information Center, P.O. Box 8057, Gaithersburg, MD 20898-8057.

Loss and Grief

When you have experienced a significant loss, you are often overwhelmed with feelings of pain and sadness. It is difficult to focus on anything outside of yourself, and your ability to concentrate is diminished. Memory problems frequently accompany grief and will lessen over time unless the mourner becomes severely depressed.

When we talk about loss and grief, most people think primarily of death. In fact, a feeling of loss may accompany many different experiences, including moving, major surgery, retirement of yourself or your spouse, vision or hearing impairment, illness of a friend or family member, changes in financial circumstances, death of a pet, marriage of a child or friend, and changes in your own health. When two or more of these experiences occur at once, the impact is greatly increased.

EXAMPLES

- Mrs. Hammerman moved into a senior citizens' building after a two-year wait. She had been looking forward to having less responsibility and meeting new people but was surprised at how often she longed for her old home and neighbors. At the same time, she found herself forgetting appointments and family birthdays. She became more and more worried and finally went to see her doctor. After doing some tests, the doctor assured her that she wasn't losing her memory. He explained to Mrs. Hammerman that even a move you want to make may cause a lot of sadness, which can temporarily affect your memory.

- Mr. Miller had been ready to retire for several years when the day finally arrived. He looked forward to sleeping late, having no boss to answer to, and spending time in his basement workshop. However, he was surprised to discover that he often felt sad and at loose ends. He also noticed that he was forgetting things. With his wife's encouragement, he volunteered to deliver Meals on Wheels to shut-ins and began a drawing class. As he felt more useful, his sadness diminished, along with much of his forgetfulness.

Additional Example *(Loss and Grief)*

Ken had been dating Josephine for a year and a half. He thought things were going well and planned on a future with her. After the holidays, Josephine told him that she hadn't been happy in their relationship for a while and that she wanted to stop seeing him. Ken initially was very angry and told himself he was better off without her. As days passed, he found himself tearful and overwhelmed. He couldn't pay attention to his work and forgot his grandson's birthday party. He suddenly felt like his mind was old and decrepit. He wondered if he was losing his memory, but he didn't know what to do about it. After several months passed, he realized that he was feeling better and that his memory was better, as well. With the lessening of Ken's grief, his memory returned to normal.

Inactivity

Lack of Mental Stimulation

The old adage "Use it or lose it" is often applied to memory functioning. Although the evidence is not all in, keeping mentally active and using memory skills may enhance your ability to remember. Some examples of mental stimulation include:

- attending an adult education class
- participating in a discussion group
- doing crossword puzzles
- playing bridge, chess, or Trivial Pursuit
- answering "Jeopardy" or other quiz show questions
- learning to use a computer
- reading a challenging book
- using newly learned memory techniques

EXAMPLE

- Mrs. Parker has always had a great interest in current events. Although she reads the newspaper daily, she has lately found it difficult to retain the information needed to formulate her position on issues. Rather than give up, she joins the current events discussion group in her senior apartment building. She enjoys the lively discussions and finds that her memory for issues is reinforced by preparing for the group and hearing the opinions of others.

Lack of Social Interaction

Many people agree that social involvement is a major factor in maintaining or improving mental capacities. When days are uncommitted and unstructured, there is less incentive to focus and organize your thoughts, and less need to remember. In social contact you have the opportunity to talk about the week's events, which reinforces the memory of what you have done and learned.

Additional Example *(Lack of Mental Stimulation)*

Miss McClellan is eighty-seven years old and lives in Woodridge Nursing Home. She is a retired French teacher and was once very lively and talkative. In the last two years, she has withdrawn and has had little contact with the outside world. She appears quite forgetful, and the nurses expect little from her. When a young college student volunteers to visit the nursing home, the nurses match her with Miss McClellan because the student is majoring in French. At first Miss McClellan is reluctant to try to speak French, but as she becomes better acquainted with the student, she begins to try to answer her questions in French. Through the weeks of the semester, Miss McClellan grows more proficient, and the nurses are amazed that her memory for everything seems a bit sharper.

┌───┐

EXAMPLES

- You receive a letter from your daughter telling you that your granddaughter is running for class president. When your daughter calls later in the week and says, "Jenny won!" you have no idea what she is talking about. Before you assume that your memory is failing, consider the fact that you saw very few people over the week and told no one about the news. If you tell a friend about any new information you receive, you encode it more deeply and greatly increase your chances of remembering it. You have not only used more senses when talking about it (hearing and speaking the words) but also have reinforced the content by discussing it.

- You've been sick for the last month and have hardly left the house. You can't remember much about what happened yesterday or the day before. You're afraid that your memory is failing along with your health. Friends have been trying to get you to go out, but you just haven't felt like it. Finally one day you give in and go to the senior center. You discuss mutual acquaintances and the Detroit Tigers' chances of winning the World Series. These discussions give you something new to think about and trigger old memories you thought you'd forgotten. When you return home, you realize that you haven't been making an effort to learn and remember something new because every day has been the same.

└───┘

Lack of Physical Activity

Although researchers are currently investigating the connection between physical activity and memory, there is no evidence at this point that you can improve your memory through exercise. However, we know that exercise and other forms of physical activity influence factors that contribute to enhanced longevity, health, and fitness in older adults. As further research is done, we will learn more about the connection between physical activity and mental functioning.

Additional Example (*Lack of Social Interaction*)

Mr. Polanski is eighty-eight years old, lives alone, and has no relatives nearby. He suffers from severe arthritis and heart problems. He is uncomfortable and fearful when away from home. His neighbor brings in his mail each day and notices that he is becoming more forgetful. He rarely knows what day it is and has forgotten his last two doctor's appointments. When he finally sees the doctor, he has lost three pounds and looks disheveled. The doctor recommends a home health aide three times a week to provide personal care and homemaking services. After a few weeks, Mr. Polanski's neighbor notices that he seems more alert and always remembers what day it is, for he looks forward to the aide coming on Monday, Wednesday, and Friday. The interaction with the aide has improved his memory for recent events because they share conversations about daily living and current events.

Lack of Organization in Daily Life

Many instances of forgetting and losing things can be traced to a disorganized lifestyle. When you don't have a systematic way to keep track of your appointments, return things to their correct places in your home, pay bills, or store important papers in a safe place, you are more likely to be forgetful. Many people have developed a lifelong habit of being organized, while others are disorganized and have never been bothered by it. If you think that some of your instances of forgetting are due to a lack of organization, you may want to develop some new organizational habits.

EXAMPLES

- Miss Woodring complained, "I always write things down. I know about keeping lists, but then I can't find the lists." At a memory course at her senior center, she heard other participants describe the same situation. The teacher advised them to keep all lists of things to buy or do in one convenient place. Miss Woodring realized she had been making lists on odd scraps of paper and leaving them all over the house. She remedied the situation by keeping a notebook for lists on her kitchen table.

- You get a notice that your electricity is about to be turned off. You're positive that you paid the bills, but when you look in the checkbook there is no record of payment. After searching the house, you discover one bill in a kitchen drawer and another in a book you're reading. No wonder you forgot to pay the bills! Most people can't keep track of household finances without some organized system. When your bills are scattered throughout the house and you have no regular schedule for paying them, it's very easy to neglect one.

Note to the Teacher *(Lack of Organization)*

It may be helpful to have your students analyze whether some problems with memory may be related to organizational habits. If shopping lists, calendars of appointments and important dates, and lists of things to do are kept routinely and organized well, instances of forgetting can be reduced. Class members often have excellent organizational suggestions to share with one another.

✎ ASSIGNMENT ━━━━━━━━━━━━━━━━

Choose one *area of your life in which you think getting organized will help you remember.*

_____ Keeping track of my purse/keys/glasses/ _____ .

_____ Remembering everything I want at the grocery store.

_____ Remembering to send birthday cards to family and friends.

_____ Remembering to pay my bills on time.

_____ Keeping track of the scissors/tape/pencil sharpener/wrapping paper/ _____ .

_____ Remembering to put gas in the car before it's nearly empty.

_____ Remembering to put the garbage out.

_____ Your choice _____ .

Now that you have chosen one, think of a way that you can organize this area of your life so that you will remember. For example, you might put up a hook where you will always *hang your keys.*

The problem: _____

_____

_____

_____

Additional Example *(Lack of Organization)*

Mrs. Jackson has fifteen grandchildren plus numerous grandnieces and grandnephews. She likes to send two dollars and a card to each child for his or her birthday each year. She found it increasingly difficult to plan ahead for each occasion and have a card and cash on hand to send. In 1989 she forgot to send cards to four grandchildren. She didn't want this to happen again so she developed an organizational plan to allow her to give these gifts easily and routinely. Each January she purchases a card for each child and gets a supply of crisp dollar bills from the bank. She encloses the money in each card and addresses and stamps the envelopes. She clips the cards in her appointment book for the appropriate week. Everyone thinks she has an amazing memory, and she is pleased that she never forgets.

Your solution: _____

_____

_____

_____

The results: _____

_____

_____

_____

After you have accomplished this goal, why not choose another?

The problem: _____

_____

_____

_____

Your solution: _____

_____

_____

_____

The results: _____

_____

_____

_____

Fatigue

Fatigue affects your ability to concentrate and slows down the recall process. You are more likely to have trouble learning new information when you're tired. Each person should figure out which times of the day he or she is most alert and should do tasks that involve new learning at those times.

EXAMPLES

- You usually read at bedtime because it puts you to sleep. However, you can't keep the characters straight in the book you're reading, and this frustrates you. You might try reading this book when you are more alert. If you want to read before dozing off, read something you don't care about remembering.

- You have just finished the third lecture of a six-week series on health problems. You were especially looking forward to last week's lecture on diabetes because your husband has diabetes in his family. However, you realize that you remember little of the material, because you were especially tired that day. For the next lecture, you resolve to be rested and ready to take notes.

Some Physical Illnesses

Even though most older people do not develop severe memory loss, memory problems can be a sign that the body is not functioning properly. Some of the following physical illnesses can aggravate an already existing mild memory problem, or they can cause memory changes in a person who has previously exhibited no memory loss. Treatment of these conditions can result in partial or complete improvement of memory function.

- infection
- fever
- heart disease

Additional Example *(Fatigue)*

Mr. Jones is discussing the prospects of the college basketball team with a couple of friends over ice cream late one evening. He is trying to tell them what he thinks of the new recruits to this year's team. He is very frustrated because he is having trouble remembering the names of any of the players or what their high-school records were. He realizes that he is just too tired to think straight, and he wisely recognizes that after a good night's sleep, his recall will be much sharper.

- lung disease
- thyroid problems
- circulatory problems
- liver and kidney problems
- strokes
- dehydration
- low blood sugar
- diabetes
- Parkinson's disease
- anemia
- delirium

On the other hand, some types of diseases or injuries that cause damage to the brain may not be reversible. Alzheimer's disease is the major cause of irreversible memory loss (see Appendix A, p. 51). Strokes and traumatic injury to the head often cause memory problems that show improvement over time but frequently leave some irreversible changes.

If you are concerned about your memory and want to rule out a physical cause, the first step is to see your family doctor, who is familiar with your medical history. However, some physicians receive little training in assessing the mental status of older people. Therefore, it may be worthwhile to consult a physician with specific training in geriatrics who has the diagnostic skills to distinguish among a wide assortment of possible causes of memory loss. A medical assessment often includes:

- a social and medical history taken from both the patient and a relative or friend
- a thorough physical examination
- a neuropsychological exam, which is a series of tests that provide information about the thought processes
- blood tests, which are used to detect thyroid, kidney, and liver malfunctions; certain nutritional deficiencies, such as pernicious anemia or vitamin B12 deficiency; infections; and metabolic and chemical imbalances
- urinalysis, which is used to detect infections

Note to the Teacher *(Some Physical Illnesses)*

If, at the end of the course, a student continues to be concerned about memory problems, encourage him to seek a medical evaluation to determine whether a physical illness or medication might be affecting his memory. A pharmacist is also a good source of information about the side effects of medications.

Additional Example *(Some Physical Illnesses)*

Ellen Singer's son is very concerned about her forgetfulness. He continually tells her that she should try harder and thinks that she should learn some new memory techniques. He reads about a memory course in the local newspaper. He insists that his mother enroll in the course, although she is not enthusiastic. He calls the instructor to enroll her in the class and describes her problems. She repeats herself frequently and sometimes forgets that he has called. She is having trouble balancing her checkbook and has dropped out of her card game. As he paints the picture of his mother's memory problems and expresses his conviction that she could remember if she really tried, the instructor wonders if Mrs. Singer's memory problems may be due to a physical illness. She suggests to the son that he should go with his mother to her next medical appointment and discuss his concerns with her doctor.

Other possible tests that may be indicated include:

- CT scan (computerized axial tomogram): a special x-ray of the brain
- MRI (magnetic resonance imaging): a procedure that painlessly scans the brain and other body parts using no radiation
- EEG (electroencephalogram): a measurement of electrical activity (brain waves) in the brain
- lumbar puncture (spinal tap): an analysis of spinal fluid that can detect malignancies, neurosyphilis, and certain infections

---
EXAMPLE

- When Cathy, the house cleaner, arrived at Mrs. Thompson's apartment for her weekly visit, she found Mrs. Thompson in bed and quite confused. When Cathy asked her if she had had breakfast, Mrs. Thompson said she wasn't sure. Also, she could not remember Cathy's name or exactly why Cathy was there. Since Mrs. Thompson had never been so confused in the past, Cathy called a neighbor, who decided that Mrs. Thompson should go to the emergency room. The physicians at the hospital discovered that she had a serious urinary tract infection and admitted her to the hospital. When Mrs. Thompson's infection cleared up, her confusion disappeared, and she returned home feeling mentally and physically well.

For more information on Alzheimer's disease, see p. 51.

Some Medications

Some medications can make you feel drowsy or unfocused. They can slow down your recall and make it hard to concentrate. Many older people are taking too many medications or are incorrectly taking what has been prescribed. Both prescription and nonprescription medications can be the cause of confusion or the source of a memory problem. It's important to ask your doctor or pharmacist about all of your medica-

Additional Example (Some Medications)

Professor Lee has recently been diagnosed as having high blood pressure. His doctor prescribes a common medication to lower his blood pressure. After several weeks Professor Lee notices that his mind seems foggy and his memory doesn't seem as sharp as it used to. He returns to his doctor and asks if the new medication might be causing these problems. His doctor acknowledges that medications for high blood pressure can cause confusion or memory problems. He tells Professor Lee that he must continue treating his high blood pressure but agrees to prescribe a different medication. He asks Professor Lee to schedule a return visit in two weeks. At that time, the nurse informs Professor Lee that his blood pressure is under good control. He is pleased because he feels that his memory is less affected by this new medication.

tions and their side effects. Also make sure that you keep a record of every medication you are currently taking and keep all medical professionals, including your pharmacist, advised of this record.

Usually confusion or a memory problem develops within a couple of days after a person starts to take a medication, but sometimes these problems occur with a medication that has been taken for a long time. Because the brain of an older person is more sensitive to the chemicals in medications, even a previously well tolerated medication may cause problems. Any time there is a memory problem or confusion, medicines should be considered as possible causes. If the medication is the source of the problem, the confusion or memory problem will improve after the person has stopped taking the medication—usually over several days, though for some medicines the full improvement may take several months. However, a person should stop taking a prescription medicine only if a doctor advises that action.

No one can predict who will experience this type of bad effect from a medication. Memory problems or confusion may be caused by just one drug or by the combination of several. The people most at risk for memory problems from medicines are those with low body weight, those who have had a sudden change in health, those taking many medicines, those with a history of drug allergies, and those with a decrease in kidney or liver function. (This section is adapted from "Medications Causing Confusion," by Leslie Shimp, B.S., Pharm. D., Associate Professor of Pharmacy, University of Michigan, Ann Arbor, Michigan.)

--- EXAMPLE ---

• Mr. Romano has been feeling quite tired, a bit foggy, and forgetting more than he used to. His neighbor suggests that he see his family doctor for consultation. Dr. Brown takes a complete history, including a review of medications. She discovers that Mr. Romano has begun to take over-the-counter antihistamines to control his seasonal allergies, along with the sleeping pills that she had prescribed at the last visit. Dr. Brown recognizes that the combination of the two drugs may be causing Mr. Romano's fatigue and memory problems. She prescribes a shorter acting sleeping pill, so that

Supplementary Material *(Some Medications)*

The older individual is more susceptible to the deleterious effects of medications than the younger one. Several factors may contribute to this increased susceptibility. A possible increase in permeability of the blood-brain barrier can make an older person more sensitive to the chemicals in medications. Renal and hepatic clearance diminish with age, possibly leading to higher serum and tissue concentrations and prolonged duration of drug action. In addition, the older person often has greater exposure to medications; a subset of the elderly takes multiple medications due to the presence of several conditions or diseases.

Frequently, the first sign of an adverse drug reaction in an older person is a change in mental function. These changes may include: confusion, disorientation, impaired memory or judgment, inability to concentrate, agitation, psychosis, or depression. Unfortunately, these changes are too often attributed to the aging process.

Both prescription and nonprescription drugs can be the cause of confusion and memory impairment. Usually, adverse effects appear within a couple of days after the person has started the medication. However, there are instances in which they can occur with a drug that has been taken for a long time or has been previously tolerated.

Factors that can influence the incidence of confusion are: combinations of medications (even though it can be caused by just one medication); incorrect usage of a medication; low body weight; sudden changes in health; history of drug allergies; and decrease in kidney and liver function.

If a person is confused, some of the first questions that should be asked are: What medications is the person taking? Are the symptoms constant or do they occur at a certain time? Did the symptoms appear after a specific medication(s) was started or before?

(From "Medications Causing Confusion in the Elderly Patient," Leslie Shimp, Pharm. D., Associate Professor of Pharmacy, University of Michigan, and Frances M. Rodriguez-Cintron, Pharm. D. candidate, University of Michigan.)

this medication will be out of Mr. Romano's system during the daytime. She also substitutes a nonsedating allergy medication for the antihistamine. Mr. Romano finds that, over time, his memory improves with this combination of medications.

Vision and Hearing Problems

An older person with vision or hearing problems often blames his memory if he can't recall information or experiences. In fact, the problem may not be in the memory at all. When the visual impression is not seen well or the sound is not heard clearly, the information will not be recorded correctly. It is important to admit when you can't see or hear adequately and ask others to speak up or make themselves and their material visible. Frequent vision and auditory testing is necessary to insure that you're getting the aids you need. Vision and hearing abilities can change dramatically, and new technology is continually being developed that may compensate for losses.

EXAMPLES

• Your neighbor suggests that you call a realtor whose name is Abbott. When you call the realty company, you ask for Mr. Babcock. The problem here may not be your memory; your neighbor may have mumbled, or you may have trouble hearing. If you want to remember something correctly, ask the person to repeat it, spell it, or even write it down.

• At the doctor's office, the receptionist gives you an insurance form to complete at home. "Just sign in these three places, and mail it off," she says, pointing to three blanks. When you get home, you are confused by all the blank spaces and say, "I've already forgotten what she told me." However, the problem may not be in your memory. You may not have seen the spaces she pointed to. Next time, ask her to mark the spaces with a red *X*.

Note to the Teacher *(Vision and Hearing Problems)*

Most people have more trouble hearing in a group setting than in an individual interaction. Background noise and mumbled voices can make it difficult for students to hear the needed information. The instructor should make it clear from the beginning that remembering is dependent on hearing clearly. Encourage students to speak up or cup an ear if the teacher or another student is speaking too softly or too quickly.

Additional Example *(Vision and Hearing Problems)*

Pauline Barnett rages at her husband, Ted, saying "You never remember anything I tell you." He feels confused and remorseful and vows to try harder to remember. At the local health fair, both Pauline and Ted take advantage of the free hearing screenings. They are surprised to learn that Ted has a significant hearing impairment in one ear. After he gets a hearing aid, Pauline is pleased to discover that with improved hearing he is paying better attention and is remembering more of what she says.

Alcohol

Alcohol can affect your memory in two different ways: First, many people find that they are less able to tolerate alcohol as they grow older; two drinks may have been tolerated well in the past but are now too much. The effects of alcohol are more dependent on the amount consumed in one drinking occasion than on how often a person takes a drink. As far as memory is concerned, there is a greater effect on the brain if you have four drinks in one night than if you have one drink on each of four nights. Second, long-term abuse of alcohol can cause irreversible memory loss.

In addition to the direct effects of alcohol on memory, alcohol consumption can cause or worsen other factors that affect your memory:

- Depression: Alcohol acts as a depressant on the central nervous system.
- Nutritional status: Alcohol provides calories without nutritional content. Some people who drink excessively fail to eat an adequate diet.

Poor Nutrition

There is still a great deal to be learned about how nutrition affects memory, but we know that a well-balanced diet contributes to overall health. Some older people eat a limited range of foods, such as toast and canned soup, a diet that can lead to a deficiency of needed nutrients. Fresh fruits and vegetables, whole-grain cereals and breads, and low-fat dairy foods or meat should be eaten daily. Small, frequent meals can be easier to prepare than traditionally larger meals and result in healthier eating habits and adequate intake of calories. Maintaining the appropriate body weight for height and age is especially important. Being either underweight or overweight can be physiologically taxing.

The use of a normal dosage multivitamin supplement is safe and appropriate if the reasons for the inadequate diet are not easily re-

Supplementary Material *(Poor Nutrition)*

There are nutrient-related causes of memory loss that occur more frequently among older adults. It is not certain what percentage of the aged population is undernourished or malnourished, because clear nutritional standards have yet to be established for older adults. Some experts estimate that from 30 to 50 percent of older adults may be undernourished or malnourished. In addition to eating less and absorbing less of what they eat, older adults can also suffer from dental problems, loneliness, depression, physical disability, or fatigue, all factors that can make it more challenging to eat a well-balanced diet. If any of these factors is applicable, it should be addressed, because it may put the older adult at a higher risk of memory impairment.

Severe vitamin or mineral deficiencies, including deficiencies of thiamine (B1), niacin (B3), cobalamin (B12), folate, and zinc, are known to cause to reversible dementia or memory impairment. Severe deficiencies are rare among healthy older adults, however. It is unclear whether milder cases of vitamin or mineral deficiencies, which may be more common with age, impair memory functioning. There are correlations between lower blood levels of nutrients and low cognitive scores, but a causal relationship has not been proven.

Another cause of memory loss in older adults may be increased concentrations of various nutrients in the brain, due to the age-related breakdown of the blood-brain barrier. A moderate increase in concentration of a single nutrient or the introduction of a nutrient normally absent in the brain can impair memory function without other gross manifestations. This is an excellent reason to avoid nutritional fads such as amino acid supplements (unless prescribed by a health care provider for a medical reason), because an older adult may be at greater risk of side effects.

Choline (a vitamin) and lecithin (a source of choline found in the human body and various foods) have been touted as supplements that improve memory. Choline is a component of an essential brain neurotransmitter involved in long-term memory. People suffering from dementia appear to be deficient in this neurotransmitter. Research is being conducted to determine whether choline supplements improve memory function. Animal

medied. Megadoses of vitamins or minerals are not safe and should not be taken unless prescribed by a health care provider.

Older adults have increased sensitivity to caffeine, nicotine, and alcohol. They should be used in moderation or avoided altogether.

Community nutrition programs can help older adults maintain healthy eating habits. Eating with others is a very important part of mealtime for many people. Many cities and towns have programs for seniors that offer meals and fellowship in communal settings. Outreach programs can take older adults shopping for food, and homemaker services can help prepare meals in the home. For those who are homebound, there are programs that deliver meals to older adults, such as Meals on Wheels. (Courtesy of nutrition consultant Kate Jones Share, M.S., Clinical Nutritionist.)

For a nutrition checklist, see p. 55.

studies have been encouraging, but clinical trials with human beings have been disappointing. It is not likely that such supplements would be helpful for people suffering from normal lapses of memory. Because there are side effects with supplementation, choline or lecithin should not be taken unless prescribed by a physician. (Courtesy Kate Jones Share, M.S., Clinical Nutritionist.)

✎   ASSIGNMENT ━━━━━━━━━━━━━━━━━━━━━━━━━━━━━

Now that we've explained how different factors affect memory, you can evaluate which factors might be affecting you.

	Never	Sometimes	Always
1. Problems with attention	——	——	——
2. Negative expectations	——	——	——
3. Stress	——	——	——
4. Anxiety	——	——	——
5. Depression	——	——	——
6. Loss and grief	——	——	——
7. Inactivity	——	——	——
8. Lack of organization	——	——	——
9. Fatigue	——	——	——
10. Physical illness	——	——	——
11. Medication	——	——	——
12. Vision problems	——	——	——
13. Hearing problems	——	——	——
14. Alcohol	——	——	——
15. Poor nutrition	——	——	——

At this point, you might want to reread the information on the factors that pertain to you. Some of them may require professional treatment by a physician or counselor, while others can be lessened by changes in your environment or lifestyle. Almost everyone can improve memory skills by learning to use memory improvement techniques, so continue reading and consider which of the following techniques will be most useful in improving your memory.

EXERCISE: FACTORS THAT AFFECT MEMORY

True/False. Circle the answer.

T   F   1. Problems with vision or hearing can affect your memory.

T   F   2. Memory recall can be affected by emotional factors.

T   F   3. Poor memory is often due to poor observation.

T   F   4. Negative expectations have no effect on memory performance.

T   F   5. Memory problems rarely indicate the need to see a doctor.

T   F   6. Problems with your health can cause increased forgetting.

T   F   7. Only major stress will affect your memory.

T   F   8. Even if you're looking forward to a change of residence, you may notice some memory problems after you move.

T   F   9. Once your memory begins to get worse, it will never improve.

T   F   10. Increasing activity, through mental stimulation, social interaction, or physical exercise, may benefit memory.

See p. 96 for answers.

Appendix A: Alzheimer's Disease

The following material is reprinted by permission of the Alzheimer's Disease and Related Disorders Associated Inc., 919 North Michigan Avenue, Suite 1000, Chicago, Illinois 60611-1676.

What Is Alzheimer's Disease?

Alzheimer's disease (AD) is a progressive, degenerative disease that attacks the brain and results in impaired memory, thinking, and behavior. It affects an estimated 4 million American adults.

AD usually has a gradual onset. Problems remembering recent events and difficulty performing familiar tasks are early symptoms. Additionally, the Alzheimer patient may experience confusion, personality change, behavior change, impaired judgment, and difficulty finding words, finishing thoughts, or following directions. How quickly these changes occur will vary from person to person, but the disease eventually leaves its victims totally unable to care for themselves.

What Is the Difference between Alzheimer's and Senility?

Increasing public awareness of Alzheimer's disease and its devastating effects is causing many older adults and Alzheimer family members to fear that forgotten names or misplaced keys may be early signs of Alzheimer's.

Until recently, an older person who was forgetful and had difficulty caring for himself was labeled "senile." "Senility" was considered a normal part of aging.

The symptoms of "senility" are now described by the term "dementia." Health care professionals recognize that when memory loss interferes with daily activities, it is not normal and is most likely the result of a disease.

Dementia is not a normal part of aging. This is because its symptoms, which include difficulties with language, learning, thinking, and reasoning, as well as memory loss, eventually become severe enough to interfere with a person's work and social life.

Although Alzheimer's disease is the most common form of irreversible dementia, some forms of dementia are curable. Keep in mind, however, that the majority of adults over the age of 65 do not develop any form of dementia.

What Is "Normal" Memory Loss?

At some time, everyone forgets her keys or where the car is parked or the name of an acquaintance. Everyone forgets things as she goes about daily activities. Usually, we don't think anything of such brief memory lapses. Often, what has been forgotten is something of little importance and eventually the information is remembered.

Although most of us expect our bodies and our reflexes to slow down with age, physicians now recognize that many healthy individuals are also less able to remember certain types of information as they get older. Health care professionals use the term "age-associated memory impairment" (AAMI) to describe minor memory difficulties that come with age.

AAMI is neither progressive nor disabling, whereas some dementias are both. AAMI is often most noticeable when the individual is under pressure. Once the person is relaxed, he is able to remember the forgotten material without difficulty.

No "treatment" for age-associated memory loss has been developed. However, writing reminders and lists, repeating messages or names out loud, allowing more time to remember, and using association to remember names may be helpful.

In addition to AAMI, minor memory difficulties may be caused by distraction, fatigue, grief, depression, stress, illness, medication, alcohol, vision or hearing loss, lack of concentration, or an attempt to remember too many details at once.

In general, it may be beneficial to cut back on alcohol, eat well-balanced meals, and make sure that medications are being taken as prescribed and are not themselves causing problems.

Recognizing Dementia

How can you tell if memory loss is more serious than age-associated memory impairment?

Dementia is progressive. AAMI may remain unchanged for years.

Most individuals with AAMI can compensate for memory loss with reminders and notes. However, memory loss associated with dementia will begin to interfere with the normal activities of daily life. In addition, dementia will affect more than memory.

For instance, Alzheimer's disease affects the ability to use words, work with figures, solve problems, and use reasoning and judgment. Alzheimer's disease also may result in changes in mood and personality.

When "forgetfulness" starts to affect the ability to carry on daily activities, it is cause for concern. Even in advanced old age, memory loss that interferes with everyday life is not normal. It may indicate a form of dementia, and the individual should undergo a complete evaluation to find out the cause.

At this time, Alzheimer's disease cannot be cured. Related disorders such as multi-infarct dementia, Parkinson's disease, Huntington's disease, and Creutzfeldt-Jakob disease, also involve irreversible dementia.

Equally important to remember, though, are the many *reversible* causes of dementia—depression, nutritional and vitamin deficiencies, drug intoxication and interaction, thyroid imbalances, some infections, blood chemistry imbalances, tumors, some blood clots, normal pressure hydrocephalus, and excessive pressure in the brain from spinal fluid.

Getting a Diagnosis of Alzheimer's Disease

At this time, there is no single diagnostic test for Alzheimer's disease. To rule out other causes of dementia symptoms requires a complete medical, neurologic, and psychiatric evaluation, as well as neuropsychological tests. A complete history from the patient's family, including a description of the symptoms and progression, also is very valuable.

For more information on the symptoms of Alzheimer's and the necessary diagnostic tests, contact the Alzheimer's Association Chapter nearest you. The Chapter members may be able to refer you to appropriate local medical resources. Call the Association's toll-free number for the Chapter nearest you: 1-800-272-3900 (TDD: 312-335-8882).

What Is the Difference between AAMI and Alzheimer's Disease?

Activity	Alzheimer Patient	Age-Associated Memory Impairment Patient
Forgets	whole experience	parts of an experience
Remembers later	rarely	often
Follows written or spoken directions	gradually unable	usually able
Able to use notes	gradually unable	usually able
Able to care for self	gradually unable	usually able

Source: Derived from the book *Care of Alzheimer's Patients: A Manual for Nursing Home Staff,* by Lisa P. Gwyther.

Further Reading

Steps to Choosing a Physician, Action Series, Alzheimer's Association, 1991.

The 36-Hour Day: A Guide to Caring for Persons with Alzheimer's Disease and Related Dementing Illnesses, by Nancy L. Mace and Peter V. Rabins, M.D. Baltimore: Johns Hopkins University Press, 1991 (revised edition).

Understanding Alzheimer's Disease, edited by Miriam K. Aronson, Ed.D. New York: Scribner's, 1988.

All publications are available from the Alzheimer's Association national office and Chapters.

Appendix B: Nutrition

The following information is reprinted by permission of the Nutrition Screening Initiative, 2626 Pennsylvania Avenue N.W., Suite 301, Washington, DC 20037. The Nutrition Screening Initiative is a project of the American Academy of Family Physicians, the American Dietetic Association, and National Council on the Aging, Inc., and is funded in part by a grant from Ross Laboratories, a Division of Abbot Labs.

Determine Your Nutritional Health

The Warning Signs of poor nutritional health are often overlooked. Use this checklist to find out if you or someone you know is at nutritional risk. Read the statements below. Circle the number in the yes column for those that apply to you or someone you know. For each yes answer, score the number in the box. Total your nutritional score.

	Yes
I have an illness or condition that made me change the kind and/or amount of food I eat.	2
I eat fewer than 2 meals per day.	3
I eat few fruits or vegetables, or milk products.	2
I have 3 or more drinks of beer, liquor, or wine almost every day.	2
I have tooth or mouth problems that make it hard for me to eat.	2
I don't always have enough money to buy the food I need.	4
I eat alone most of the time.	1
I take 3 or more different prescribed or over-the-counter drugs a day.	1
Without wanting to, I have lost or gained 10 pounds in the last 6 months.	2
I am not always physically able to shop, cook and/or feed myself.	2
Total	_____

Total Your Nutritional Score. If it's—

0–2   Good! Recheck your nutritional score in 6 months.

3–5   You are at moderate nutritional risk. See what can be done to improve your eating habits and lifestyle. Your office on aging, senior nutrition program, senior citizens center, or health department can help. Recheck your nutritional score in 3 months.

6 or more   You are at high nutritional risk. Bring this checklist the next time you see your doctor, dietitian, or other qualified health or social service professional. Talk with them about any problems you may have. Ask for help to improve your nutritional health.

Remember that warning signs suggest risk, but do not represent diagnosis of any condition. Read on to learn more about the Warning Signs of poor nutritional health.

The Nutrition Checklist is based on the Warning Signs described below. Use the word *DETERMINE* to remind you of the Warning Signs.

DISEASE

Any disease, illness, or chronic condition which causes you to change the way you eat, or makes it hard for you to eat, puts your nutritional health at risk. Four out of five adults have chronic diseases that are affected by diet. Confusion or memory loss that keeps getting worse is estimated to affect one out of five or more of older adults. This can make it hard to remember what, when, or if you've eaten. Feeling sad or depressed, which happens to about one in eight older adults, can cause big changes in appetite, digestion, energy level, weight, and well-being.

EATING POORLY

Eating too little and eating too much both lead to poor health. Eating the same foods day after day or not eating fruit, vegetables, and milk products daily will also cause poor nutritional health. One in five adults skips meals daily. Only 13% of adults eat the minimum amount of fruit and vegetables needed. One in four older adults drinks too much alcohol. Many health problems become worse if you drink more than one or two alcoholic beverages per day.

TOOTH LOSS/MOUTH PAIN

A healthy mouth, teeth, and gums are needed to eat. Missing, loose, or rotten teeth or dentures which don't fit well or cause mouth sores make it hard to eat.

ECONOMIC HARDSHIP

As many as 40% of older Americans have incomes of less than $6,000 per year. Having less—or choosing to spend less—than $25–30 per week for food makes it very hard to get the foods you need to stay healthy.

REDUCED SOCIAL CONTACT

One-third of all older people live alone. Being with people daily has a positive effect on morale, well-being, and eating.

MULTIPLE MEDICINES

Many older Americans must take medicines for health problems. Almost half of older Americans take multiple medicines daily. Growing old may change the way we respond to drugs. The more medicines you take, the greater the chance for side effects such as increased or decreased appetite, change in taste, constipation, weakness, drowsiness, diarrhea, nausea, and others. Vitamins or minerals when taken in large doses act like drugs and can cause harm. Alert your doctor to everything you take.

INVOLUNTARY WEIGHT LOSS/GAIN

Losing or gaining a lot of weight when you are not trying to do so is an important warning sign that must not be ignored. Being overweight or underweight also increases your chance of poor health.

NEEDS ASSISTANCE IN SELF CARE

Although most older people are able to eat, one of every five has trouble walking, shopping, and buying and cooking food, especially as they get older.

ELDER YEARS ABOVE AGE 80

Most older people lead full and productive lives. But as age increases, risk of frailty and health problems increases. Checking your nutritional health regularly makes good sense.

4 Memory Improvement Techniques

Everyone has to make choices about what is important to remember. No one remembers everything. Once you have determined that you want to improve your memory in a particular area, you can select a strategy for change. In this chapter we describe sixteen techniques for improving your memory. They are:

- association
- visualization
- active observation
- elaboration
- written reminders
- auditory reminders
- environmental change
- self-instruction
- story method
- chunking
- first letter cues
- create a word
- categorization
- search your memory
- alphabet search
- review

59

There are two general types of memory improvement techniques: those that occur internally (within the mind) and those that involve the external environment. Although there are only three external techniques included in this book (written reminders, auditory reminders, and environmental change), a large proportion of the memory tasks of older adults is accomplished by the use of these techniques. Older adults can be encouraged to expand their repertoires to include the use of internal techniques. It is challenging and satisfying to be able to remember things within one's mind. It is also the case that external techniques are not always available or appropriate for remembering certain things.

Because the expectation of students in a memory improvement class is that they will learn techniques that will help them improve their memories, it is frustrating for them to wait until the end of the course to learn those techniques. Thus, we intersperse the teaching of the techniques throughout the course sessions. On pp. 103–5, we have presented a suggested sequence for a memory course. However, you may choose to change the order of the techniques based on the memory problems presented by your students. When teaching internal techniques we always begin with association (p. 61). Understanding how association works is essential to understanding many of the other internal techniques.

Some of these techniques involve cues in your environment, such as notes, lists, signs, or buzzers. Other techniques improve the way you encode the information you want to remember so that you can retrieve it more easily. Some of these techniques will be familiar; others will seem strange. It is difficult to know which ones will be useful for you without trying them several times. Look for chances to experiment.

We have found that it is fun and rewarding to figure out a way to remember and to succeed. We believe that there is a tool for remembering almost anything. However, in some cases you may decide that the effort needed is not worth the benefit gained. Recognize that the choice is yours to make.

Here's the best way to use these memory improvement techniques:

1. Choose something specific that you want to remember.
2. Review the possible techniques and select one.
3. Try the technique. (If it works, congratulations!)
4. If your chosen technique does not work, try something else.
5. Don't feel defeated if some things are particularly hard to remember. Ask yourself if it really matters anyway.

WHAT ARE SOME GENERAL STRATEGIES FOR IMPROVING MEMORY?

Although there are many techniques for remembering specific kinds of information, there are four strategies that can be used whenever you want to encode almost any kind of new information securely so that it is available for retrieval.

The four general strategies for improving memory are:

Association: Associate what you want to remember with what you know.

Visualization: Visualize a picture of what you want to remember.

Active observation: Actively observe and think about what you want to remember.

Elaboration: Elaborate on the details of the information you want to remember.

People who have excellent memories use these strategies on a daily basis. It will take thought and practice, but if you can incorporate these strategies into everyday life, you will have a better memory.

Associate What You Want to Remember with What You Know

Association is the process of forming mental connections between what you want to remember and what you already know. Although many associations are made automatically, the conscious creation of associations is an excellent strategy for encoding new information. Once you make an association, repeating it several times either in your head or aloud will help you remember.

This technique can be used to remember:

- the name of your new neighbor
- the street where your friend lives
- the title of a movie you want to recommend
- whether to turn right or left to get to the restaurant
- the number of the bus to your friend's house

EXAMPLES

- *Mr. Miller:* My daughter asked me to pick up a special kind of crackers called Cheese Delight at the grocery store. I wanted to see if I could remember it without writing it down, so I worked on figuring out an association. Crackers and cheese have always been a good combination to me, so I could remember the "cheese" part easily. The "delight" part was a little more difficult. I thought about

Additional Examples *(Associate What You Want to Remember with What You Know)*

You may have heard of a way to remember whether to turn a jar lid or a screw to the left or the right to tighten or loosen. Many people say to themselves "Lefty, loosey; righty, tighty." This phrase connects the task of loosening and tightening with the familiar directions of left and right and associates them in such a way that they are well encoded and easily recalled.

Millie Walker has begun taking a new medicine, Prozac, for depression. Occasionally a friend or relative will ask her for its name, and she can never remember. She complains about it to her daughter Sue, who says, "We can come up with a way to remember the name. Let's analyze the way the word sounds or what it means." Millie says, "Well, I can remember the first part. It reminds me of pro and con, and I hope it's working *for* me, not against." Sue says, "Zac doesn't mean anything, but it's easy to rhyme. Pro*zac* will put you *back* on *track*." They laugh and feel proud. Working together makes this memory task easier and more fun.

how delighted I would be if I could succeed at this task and registered the word and feeling in my mind. When I got to the store and looked at the countless kinds of crackers, the Cheese Delight box jumped right out at me and I thought, "Association really works!"

- *Mr. Cavender:* I have two cars that have gas caps on opposite sides, and I could never remember which was which. Each time I went to fill up, I had to ponder which way to approach the gas pumps, and I felt aggravated. I decided to consciously find an association that would register the information once and for all. I first noted that the gas cap was on the left side of my tan car. Now, what could I associate with left? I thought about the fact that this car is lighter in color than my black car, so I could associate the "l" in *light* and *left*. For several weeks, each time I drove into the gas station, I said to myself, "In this light car, the gas cap is on the left."

- *Ms. Spencer:* I had a new neighbor whose name was Marsha. For some reason I had a hard time remembering her name. I had learned about association in a memory course and decided to try it. After looking carefully at Marsha, I noticed she had white, fluffy hair. I decided that I could remember her name by associating Marsha with marshmallow. Each time I saw her, I associated her hair with a big marshmallow and said to myself, "Marshmallow Marsha."

EXERCISE: ASSOCIATION

Create an association between the following items of new information and something you already know.

1. You must remember to take the entrance marked "west" on the expressway to get to the doctor's office.

   _____

   _____

   _____

2. You want to remember the year your grandson was born, which is 1968.

   _____

   _____

   _____

3. You want to remember Rose Campbell's name.

   _____

   _____

   _____

4. You want to remember the name "Turner Medical Clinic."

   _____

   _____

   _____

See p. 96 for possible answers.

Visualize a Picture of What You Want to Remember

You have often heard that a picture is worth a thousand words. Visualization is the process of consciously creating an image in your mind of a task, a number, a name, a word, or an abstract thought. If you take the time to translate words into a meaningful picture and hold that picture in your mind for a few seconds, you are more likely to remember the name, the task, or the thought.

This technique can be used to remember:

- items you need to buy at the grocery store
- the route from the airport terminal to where you parked your car
- the laundry basket you want to bring up from the basement
- the name of a new breakfast cereal that you want to try
- the punch line of a joke you recently heard

EXAMPLES

- *Mrs. Pinelle:* When I was shopping last month, I saw such a beautiful dress in the window of a new store called Toshiros. I knew I'd never remember the name of this shop because it was unfamiliar to me, and I didn't know what it meant. When I repeated the name over to myself, I imagined a big hairy toe and a razor getting ready to shear the hair off—"Toe-shear-o."

- *Ms. Barton:* I love to tell my friends about my favorite restaurant. It's so expensive that I can only go there once a year, so I don't see the name very often. It's called Justine's, which is a name I have trouble remembering. However, I do know that they have a young chef, so I imagine a very youthful face with a big chef's hat on, and think "Why, he's 'just a teen.'"

- *Mr. Simon:* I get so angry when I get up from my chair, put on my coat, walk to the back of my yard to get something from the garage, then forget what I went to get. After taking a memory course, I found out that if I take the time to picture what I'm getting up

Additional Example *(Visualize a Picture of What You Want to Remember)*

Mr. Kim is taking a memory improvement course through his local adult education department. The instructor teaches the technique of visualization. Mr. Kim decides to practice this technique to remember the three errands he has to run one afternoon. He plans to go to the library, to the hardware store, and to the jeweler to have his watch fixed. He thinks about the most efficient route to follow in completing his errands. He visualizes himself driving down the parkway past the swimming pool to the mall where the jeweler and the hardware store are located. He pictures himself buying a new rake and handing his watch to the jeweler. Next he imagines himself leaving the mall and driving through the busy downtown area to the library. He visualizes himself checking out a colorful book on gardening. He realizes that he has fixed his route and individual errands well in his mind in under a minute. He is pleasantly surprised that this technique is so easy and useful.

Exercise for In-Class Use *(Visualize a Picture of What You Want to Remember)*

Experts believe that we lose the tendency to spontaneously create mental images as we grow older. Your students may be reluctant to attempt the technique of visualization if it appears to be more work than it is worth. If you demonstrate the power of this technique to your students in class, they may be more likely to try it on their own.

Tell students that you will read them a four-sentence story and will then ask them how many facts they can remember without using paper or pencil. Read Scenario 1 slowly, giving students time to use any memory technique they may choose, but give them no instructions to do so. Afterward, have them list as many facts as they can remember about the story. Next, discuss the technique of visualization and instruct students to create mental images as you slowly read Scenario 2. Then have students list as many facts as they can remember from the second story.

Next, ask students to discuss which techniques they used to remember the facts from both scenarios. Were they able to visualize either or both

for, I can remember most of the time. Just yesterday, I wanted the flashlight from my car. I remembered it as blue, and I envisioned myself using it to look in the attic. When I got to the car, I had no trouble remembering what I went for.

EXERCISE: VISUALIZATION

Create a visual image to help you remember the following:

1. Mrs. Hammerman's name

_____

_____

_____

2. An echogram

_____

_____

_____

3. Parkinson's disease

_____

_____

_____

4. Lane 5B in a parking lot

_____

_____

_____

stories? Did visualization help them to remember? Were other techniques as effective?

Some students may use visualization routinely, while others may depend on pure rote memory. For those who do not spontaneously create mental images, this exercise can demonstrate the power of visualization for remembering.

Scenario 1

A grandmother and grandfather and their two pre-school-aged grandchildren went for a drive in their red van on a rainy day. They passed a fruit stand and decided to turn back to buy some sweet cherries and squash. They drove to a diner and had turkey dinner with corn and biscuits. They returned home on a gravel road, where they were chased by a barking dog.

There are 22 facts in scenario 1:

grandmother	rain	corn
grandfather	fruit stand	biscuits
two	turn back	home
pre-school-aged	sweet cherries	gravel road
grandchildren	squash	chased
drive	diner	barking
red	turkey	dog
van		

Now go on to Scenario 2.

5. To buy a new windshield wiper blade while at the gas station

_____

_____

_____

See page 97 for possible answers.

Actively Observe and Think about What You Want to Remember

It is often difficult to remember things that you haven't observed clearly or with much interest. Active observation is the process of consciously paying attention to the details of what you see, hear, or read. By using active observation you can find meaning and vibrancy in a photograph, a new face, a nature scene, a conversation, an occurrence on the street, or a piece of artwork. Active observation contrasts with a passive attitude of letting life go on around you without much thought or interest. To actively observe a subject, think about the meaning of the subject, how you feel about it, how it affects you, and whether you *want* to remember it. Ask yourself questions that will reinforce its meaning. One key to remembering is being interested.

This technique can be used to remember:

- the design of a quilt you saw in a store
- how to play a new game that your grandchild is teaching you
- the faces of people you see in the hallway of your apartment complex
- the difference between a fir tree and a juniper

Scenario 2

A lifeguard at a rocky beach drove to work on his silver motorcycle. He changed from blue jeans to a green bathing suit and put his whistle around his neck. He hollered at three teen-agers who were out too far to come closer to shore. At sunset, his blonde girlfriend brought him a hot dog, a Coke, and some potato chips.

There are 22 facts in scenario 2:

lifeguard	bathing suit	come closer
rocky	whistle	sunset
beach	neck	blonde
silver	hollered	girlfriend
motorcycle	three	hot dog
changed clothes	teen-agers	Coke
blue jeans	too far out	potato chips
green		

Additional Examples *(Actively Observe and Think about What You Want to Remember)*

If your daughter takes you to a new doctor's office for a first visit and you plan to drive yourself for the second visit, you will need to actively observe the landmarks and road signs. You may have noticed that if you ride passively in a car, you are often unable to re-create your route.

If you want to distinguish between a sparrow and a wren at your bird feeder, you must pay attention to the ways in which they are similar and different. Instruct yourself to note details about color, size, shape, sound, and habits. The passive observer might see two smallish brown-gray birds. The active observer will learn to differentiate between them.

┌───┐

EXAMPLES

- *Mrs. Sung:* I have very bad arthritis and am in a wheelchair. I was so depressed and bored—every day was just the same, and my memory was getting really bad. My daughter gave me a bird feeder for my birthday, and little by little I started watching the birds that came. One day I saw a bird I didn't recognize. I asked my daughter if she knew what it was. She didn't, either, but the next time she visited me, she brought a colored picture book of hundreds of birds and facts about them. When we looked up the bird, I was amazed at how many kinds there are in Michigan. That bird feeder has changed my life! I'm seeing and learning new things, and I'm surprised that I can really remember them.

- *Miss Robinson:* I parked in a large parking garage when going to Senior Power Day at the state capitol building. There were several up and down ramps on each level and no letters or numbers designating the area in which I parked. I realized that I could easily misplace my car. I carefully observed the route I took to the exit stairway and, when I got there, looked back to reinforce the image of the location of my car. When I returned several hours later, I had a strong memory of where my car was located and how to get there.

- *Mr. Hooper:* After taking a memory course and learning about active observation, I decided to give it a try. I went to our local museum and spent some time looking at a painting of two women by Monet. Instead of just glancing at the painting as I usually do, I looked at the details as well as the whole and asked myself some questions: Did I think it was pretty? What time of year was it? Did the women look happy or sad? What were they wearing? Was there anything especially unusual about the painting? Would I like to have it in my living room? When I left the museum, I knew that I would remember something from this trip to the museum; it would not be just the usual blur of pictures.

└───┘

Exercise for In-Class Use *(Actively Observe and Think about What You Want to Remember)*

We have found that a good way to demonstrate the effectiveness of active observation is to show two slides that depict a scene, a group of people, or an artwork. Each slide should have quite a bit of detail, color, and meaning. Give no instructions when asking students to spend one minute observing the first slide. Afterward, ask specific questions about the content of the slide designed to test students' observational skills. Next, describe the process of active observation. Ask the students to use the following guidelines that will assist their observational skills as they view the second slide for one minute.

1. What are the important details?
2. What is the mood, time of day, or season?
3. What is happening in the picture?
4. How does it relate to me?
5. Do I like what I see?
6. How am I going to remember this?

After viewing the second slide, again ask the students specific questions about the content of the slide designed to test observational skills. Most students will discover that they remember better when using active observation rather than passively looking at the slide.

People can have fun saying their answers aloud. This is not a test to see who has the best memory, just a demonstration of the powers of observation.

EXERCISE: ACTIVE OBSERVATION

Look at the picture below, consciously paying attention to the details. Ask yourself questions about the picture's meaning and its effect on you as you look at it.

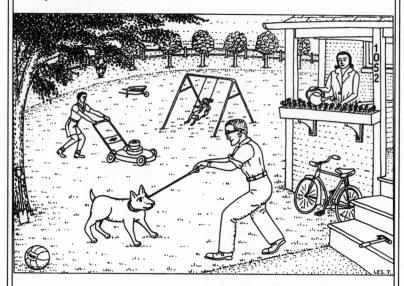

Now, cover the picture and see if you can answer these questions.

- How many people are in the picture?
- What is the boy doing?
- What is the woman doing?
- What is leaning against the house?
- What is on the steps?
- Name the items in the yard.
- What is the number on the house?
- What is the boy wearing?
- What is the man doing?

If you are able to answer all of the above questions, you have used excellent powers of observation. Take a second look, if you aren't sure of the correct answers.

Exercise for In-Class Use *(Actively Observe and Think about What You Want to Remember)*

If you do not have access to slides and a slide projector, you can provide an exercise in active observation by observing the details of the room that you are in. Have participants close their eyes and ask them to answer the following five questions about the room.

1. How many windows are there?
2. What color are the walls?
3. What sort of light fixtures are there?
4. Is there a clock in the room?
5. What does the floor look like?

Next, ask them to spend one minute looking around the room observing as much as they can. You may give guidelines for observation, as in the previous exercise using slides. Then, have the students close their eyes and respond to the following five questions.

1. Does the door open in or out?
2. Are there prints or posters on the walls?
3. What is the teacher wearing?
4. What color are the chairs?
5. What is covering the windows?

**Elaborate on the Details of the Information
You Want to Remember**

A brief, unexamined thought is very fragile and easily forgotten. When we elaborate on the details of a thought or idea, we encode it more deeply. We experience this depth of processing unintentionally when something very interesting or controversial occurs. In our minds, we comment on the occurrence; we try to understand what happened; we relate it to what we know of the situation; we ask ourselves how we feel about it. This process can be used intentionally as a strategy for encoding information we want to remember.

Try this technique if you want to remember:

- the instructions for using your new vacuum attachments
- the platforms of the two mayoral candidates
- the courses that your grandson is taking in college
- the directions to the new recreation building.

── EXAMPLES ──────────

- *Mr. Simon:* I recently purchased a new VCR, read the instructions, and tediously followed them to record my favorite TV show. The next time I tried to record a show, I couldn't remember what to do and had to reread the instruction manual. Because I wanted to be able to program my VCR in the future without referring to the manual, I was determined to encode the information well by using the technique of elaboration. I talked myself through the steps, figuring out the order and importance of each step. I translated the stilted manual directions into my own language. I repeated the steps several times to fix them in my long-term memory. I discovered that it works even better if you use this technique aloud. Even after being on vacation for three weeks, I could still remember the steps.

Additional Example *(Elaborate on the Details of the Information You Want to Remember)*

At her nutrition class, Mrs. Bradley was given brochures from her two favorite fast-food restaurants. They listed all of the menu items with descriptions of calories, salt content, and fat content. She read the brochures with interest and noticed which items would fit her diet requirements. The next time she went to one of these restaurants she was disappointed to discover that she could no longer remember which were the most nutritious items. Because she was unlikely to carry the brochures with her every time she wanted to stop for lunch, she decided to find a way to encode the information so that she could retrieve it when she wanted.

She read through the brochures to determine which items she might possibly order. She decided that each restaurant had a couple of items that suited her diet. For example, in Restaurant A, she would order a small hamburger without cheese or a chicken salad with low fat dressing; however, in Restaurant B, the chicken sandwich or a large baked potato were her best choices. She made associations between the name of the restaurants and the menu choices. She repeated the associations and visualized herself eating the food in each restaurant. She was successful in encoding this information into long-term memory well enough to recall it when needed.

- *Miss Kirby:* I took a trip of a lifetime to the Hawaiian Islands. I visited three of the islands—all of which are gorgeous, yet different from each other. I wanted to be able to tell my friends about the islands without mixing them up. I had read in the newspaper that if you elaborate on the details of what you want to remember, you will encode the information more deeply. I thought about the different physical characteristics of the island, what I did on each island, and where I stayed. I made some associations between these details and the names of the islands. For several days I repeated these details, and now I find it easy to remember.

EXERCISE: ELABORATION

Every state has a nickname by which it is known. Here are the nicknames of three states:

Minnesota: The Gopher State
Missouri: The Show Me State
Montana: The Treasure State

See if you can use elaboration to encode these states and their nicknames so that you can remember them tomorrow. When you wake up tomorrow, ask yourself if you can remember this information. If not, try elaborating on it more fully.

DO I HAVE TO REMEMBER EVERYTHING IN MY HEAD?

Although there are times when you have to rely upon your mind for remembering, most of us use external reminders to prompt us throughout our daily lives. For example, we may use an alarm clock to wake up in the morning; keep a calendar of appointments; make grocery lists; use a kitchen timer for baking cookies; and use a marked pill box. Everyone agrees that there is no need to trust our memory in these situations. If we can use something in our environment to cue us, our minds are free to think of other things. Even though the following three external techniques may be familiar to you, consider finding new ways to adapt them to your needs:

Written reminders: Write things down.

Auditory reminders: Use sound to trigger your memory.

Environmental change: Change something in your surroundings so that it jogs your memory.

Write Things Down

Although people of all ages use lists, calendars, appointment books, and notes to keep track of what they want to remember, many older people believe that written reminders shouldn't be necessary. Writing things down is one of the most useful memory tools. As you age you may need to make even greater use of written reminders for both future events and as a diary of the day's happenings.

If you are having trouble remembering the people you meet, what you read, or how you spend your day, keep all that information in one diary. On a similar note, all financial papers and bills should be kept in one place and recorded systematically.

┌─ EXAMPLES ─────────────────────────────────┐

- Keep a running list of things you need to do. As soon as you think of something, add it to the list. Keep this list in a permanent place where you can't help but notice it.

- Use an appointment book or calendar to remind yourself of up-coming events and make a habit of looking at it frequently.

- Keep a list of health questions you want to ask your physician at your next appointment. Write down instructions from the physician before you leave the office.

- Keep a diary of what has happened each day so that if you wonder whether you've written a letter or made an important phone call you can refer to the diary. Include the names of people you've met.

- Keep a list of books you want to read or have read.

- Keep a notebook where you record letters and greeting cards sent and received.

└──┘

 ASSIGNMENT ━━━━━━━━━━━━━━━━━━━━━━━━━━━

Within the next three days buy a notebook that you will use to record whatever you want to remember. Keep a record for one week.

For example:

Pd. car insurance
sent package to Jane
met new neighbor —Jack

Buy thread
Call plumber 769-1130
Watch TV special
on S. Africa 9:00

Additional Examples *(Write Things Down)*

Keep a record of the name and dosage of each medication. Include the date you began taking it.

Keep a record of each doctor's visit by date so that you can keep track of insurance reimbursement.

Make lists of people whose names you want to remember, such as neighbors, members of a social group, or children of your friends.

Keep a record of the anniversaries of events you would like to recall, such as the death of your friend's husband or child.

Record in an appointment book or favorite cookbook when you had guests to dinner and what you served them. Be sure to note any failures.

Collect take-out menus from your favorite ethnic restaurants and mark your favorite menu items so that you can recall what you have enjoyed (or disliked) in the past.

Use Sound to Trigger Your Memory

Alarm clocks and kitchen timers can be used to remind yourself of something that can't be done immediately but that must be done at a specific time. A telephone answering machine can also be used to provide an auditory cue.

EXAMPLES

- If you make a phone call and get a busy signal, set your kitchen timer to remind yourself to call again.

- If you're busy writing letters and want to be sure to leave for an appointment at a specific time, set the kitchen timer and carry it with you to your desk.

- If you are away from home and want to remember to do something when you return, leave yourself a message on your answering machine.

Change Something in Your Surroundings
So That It Jogs Your Memory

One of the best and easiest ways to remind yourself of a specific task is to change something in your environment so that you notice the change. It then serves as a cue to jog your memory. It is imperative that you make the change as soon as you think of the task.

EXAMPLES

- Put the clothes to take to the cleaners in front of the door.

- Move the telephone out of its ordinary place as a way to remind yourself to call someone later.

- Put a note on the refrigerator so that you'll see it when you eat breakfast and remember to send a card to your son.

Additional Examples *(Use Sound to Trigger Your Memory)*

Carry a small battery-operated or wind-up alarm clock in your purse or pocket to remind you to take your medicine at a particular time.

If you worry that you might lose track of time and be late to pick up your grandchild from school, use an alarm clock or kitchen timer to remind you.

- Put a note on the steering wheel to remind yourself to vote or stop at the cleaners.

- Tie a string around the handles of your purse so that you can't open it without being reminded of what you need to do.

- Put an empty box in front of the basement stairway to remind yourself to turn off the electric heater when you go upstairs.

- Change your watch or ring to the other hand; you will constantly feel it, and it will remind you of what you need to do.

When using any of these external reminders, it is crucial to avoid procrastination. As soon as you think of something you need to do in the future, choose one of these techniques and act upon it. If you think, "I'll add potatoes to my grocery list when this TV show is over," you may forget all about it ten minutes later.

EXERCISE: ENVIRONMENTAL CHANGE
Think of ways to jog your memory for the following tasks by using environmental change.

1. You want to remember to bring your lasagna pan to the senior center tomorrow.

_____

_____

_____

_____

_____

Additional Examples *(Change Something in Your Surroundings So That It Jogs Your Memory)*

If you have been disappointed by forgetting to take your camera on a vacation in the past, leave a note taped to the bottom of your suitcase to remind yourself to take your camera when you travel.

Keep a clothespin in your glove box so that you can clip it to your steering wheel on dark days as a reminder to turn off your lights when you reach your destination.

Put your old clothes for donation to the thrift shop in your car so that someday when you are in the right location, you will remember to drop them off.

Tie a string loosely around your wrist; you will constantly feel it, and it will remind you of what you need to do.

When you awaken at night with something on your mind that needs to be done, move your book from the nightstand to the top of the lamp.

2. You are out grocery shopping and want to remember to call your dentist when you get home.

_____

_____

_____

_____

3. You are at your exercise class and a friend asks you to bring a certain book to tomorrow's class.

_____

_____

_____

_____

4. You want to remember to put out the garbage tomorrow.

_____

_____

_____

_____

5. You are sitting in church and you remember that you have to stop at the store on your way home.

_____

_____

_____

_____

See p. 97 for possible solutions.

HOW CAN I AVOID WORRYING ABOUT WHETHER I HAVE DONE WHAT I INTENDED TO DO?

Many daily tasks are done automatically; we don't pay much attention to them. In order to avoid worrying about whether you have unplugged the iron, turned off the electric blanket, or locked the door, you can use the technique of *self-instruction*.

Give Yourself Verbal Instructions about What You Want to Remember

Self-instruction is the process of giving yourself mental or verbal reinforcement so that you will pay attention to what you want to remember. This technique is powerful because it focuses your attention on an act that is often done automatically and thus is easily forgotten. Use this technique to fix in your mind tasks about which you may ask yourself later, "Did I remember to do that?" As you turn off the coffeepot, say aloud to yourself, "I am now turning off the coffeepot," and you won't wonder about it later.

Sometimes you can use this technique to remind yourself to do something in the immediate future. You might need to provide more detail to reinforce your memory for a future task. As you drive to the grocery store at dusk, remind yourself aloud to turn off the lights. One sentence is not enough in this case. You might say, "I'm putting my lights on as I go to the grocery store. When I get into the parking lot at Supermart, I must remember to turn them off." You might also visualize the lights shining on the store window as you arrive, then see yourself turning them off.

Note to the Teacher *(Give Yourself Verbal Instructions about What You Want to Remember)*

People find this technique more effective if they speak aloud and use a lot of elaborative detail. For example, if you worry about whether you have locked your front door, you might say aloud, "It's Tuesday. I won't have to face an intruder because I've locked my door." Be aware that if someone says the same words every day, this technique can become so routine that it loses its power. It's important to change the story every now and then.

EXAMPLE

- *Ms. Heinz:* One thing I hoped to get out of a memory course was learning how to remember whether I put detergent in the washer. I would get upstairs and have to go back down because I was never sure whether I did it. The instructors suggested that, as I add the detergent, I say to myself, "There, I just put the soap into the washer." I gave it a try, and now I always say something aloud like, "Good, I won't have to come down here again because I just added the soap," and it really works for me.

 ASSIGNMENT ━━━━━━━━━━━━━━━━━━━━━━━━━━━━

For the rest of the day, use self-instruction whenever you perform a task that might cause you to ask later, "Did I do that?" At the end of the day look through the list below and check the ways you used this technique or might use it in the future. Notice if using this technique was helpful.

- turning off the stove/iron/coffeepot/heater
- locking the door
- turning off the car lights
- turning down the heat
- adding the laundry soap
- making a phone call
- taking medicine
- turning off the basement light/front porch light
- closing the garage door
- putting the gas cap back on the gas tank
- watering the plants
- other

ARE THERE ANY TECHNIQUES THAT COULD HELP WHEN I HAVE SEVERAL ITEMS TO REMEMBER?

It is always easier to remember fewer items than more. Look for ways to connect or combine the items so that they can be remembered collectively. You'll understand this concept when you read about the following techniques:

Story method: Devise a story that will connect things you want to remember.

Chunking: Chunk individual items into a group.

First letter cues: Group the first letters of a series of items.

Create a word: Expand random letters into a familiar word.

Categorization: Group a list of items by category.

Devise a Story That Will Connect Things You Want to Remember

The story method is the process of making up a simple, yet colorful, tale connecting items that seem to have no connection. This is a technique that many people resist because it seems either silly or too complicated. We believe that if you give it a try, you will find it amazingly effective. This technique can be used to remember:

- two phone calls that you need to make when you get home
- three things you want to tell your daughter when you call her
- three items you need to pick up at the hardware store
- two books you want to get at the library.

EXAMPLES
- You wake up in the night and start thinking of what you need to do the next day. You want to remember that you need to call your dentist, return a rug to the department store, and get an oil change for your car, but you don't want to get out of bed to make a list.

Note to the Teacher *(Are There Any Techniques That Could Help When I Have Several Items to Remember?)*

The techniques in this section may seem intimidating and too difficult, but using these techniques is helpful when you want to remember several unrelated things. Give students plenty of opportunity to practice in class. Try to make it fun and challenging so that they will give it a good try. The exercises in the guide and the in-class exercises will demonstrate clearly the power of these techniques.

You make up a story connecting these items by visualizing your dentist using a rug to keep himself warm because his car has run out of oil and is stalled.

• You think of four items that you want to buy at the drugstore: a birthday card, a sponge, a bottle of shampoo, and some film. You create a story about shampooing your hair with a sponge while signing a birthday card, and a photographer bursts in to take your photo.

EXERCISE: STORY METHOD

Make up a one- or two-sentence story connecting the following items:

1. Getting a duplicate key made, picking up a birthday cake, and going to the bank

  _____

  _____

  _____

  _____

  _____

2. Shopping for stationery, cologne, and a broom

  _____

  _____

  _____

  _____

  _____

  _____

See p. 97 for possible solutions.

Additional Examples *(Devise a Story That Will Connect Things You Want to Remember)*

You have to go to the cleaners and post office before you go home. You might make up a story about putting your pants into the mailbox and dealing with the chaos that would follow.

Eleanor wakes up one night thinking about what she has to do the next day. She has to mail a package to her sister, get a prescription refilled, and call the furnace repairman. She connects the three tasks in a brief story and creates a vivid mental image. She imagines the repairman delivering a large package of pills to her sister.

You are going to a dinner party at the home of your friend Mary. She has recently married a man who has an unusual first name. You check the invitation and note that his name is Cole. Because you are unfamiliar with that name, you are afraid that you may forget it. You decide to try the story method that you learned in your memory class. You create a story in which Mary and her Little Lamb meet Old King Cole for dinner.

Chunk Individual Items into a Group

It is easier to remember three items than seven. When you are trying to remember a group of numbers, look for ways to combine them. This technique can be used to remember:

- phone numbers
- street addresses and zip codes
- social security and driver's license numbers

EXAMPLES

- If you want to remember a local telephone number such as 764-2556, you can usually remember the prefix because it is fairly familiar. However, if you group the last four numbers into two chunks, 25 and 56, the phone number will be easier to recall.

- A driver's license or social security number may seem almost impossible to remember. However, if you learn it in chunks it will be more manageable. 343–49–4296 could be 3-43-49-42-96 or 34-34-94-29-6 or 343-494-296.

EXERCISE: CHUNKING
Memorize your driver's license number or Social Security number by chunking the individual numbers. Analyze the sequence to see which way of chunking makes the most sense.

_____

_____

_____

Additional Examples *(Chunk Individual Items into a Larger Group)*

Children remember the alphabet by grouping individual letters into chunks and reciting them to the rhythm of "Twinkle, Twinkle, Little Star":

A-B-C-D-E-F-G
H-I-J-K-LMNOP
Q-R-S
T-U-V
W-X-Y and Z
Now I've learned my ABCs
Aren't you very proud of me?

Note that this example also uses the technique of rhyming.

Since his move to a new state, Art could never remember the numbers on his license plate, 749. He decided to analyze them and see if he could divide them into chunks that made them easier to remember. He knows that 49 is divisible by 7, so by chunking the numbers into 7 and 49, it was easier to recall.

Group the First Letters of a Series of Items

This technique involves using the first letters of a list of words to form either another word or a meaningful sentence whose words begin with the same letters as the words on the list. Although this technique is hard to describe, it's easy to use. The following examples should give you the idea.

EXAMPLES

- If you want to remember the names of the five Great Lakes, you can take the first letter of each lake and create the word HOMES (Huron, Ontario, Michigan, Erie, Superior).

- If you want to remember the names of each of the presidents from Eisenhower to Clinton, you can take the first letter of each name and form a sentence that has meaning to you. One example is: "Every kid juggles nine fine china rings before class" (Eisenhower, Kennedy, Johnson, Nixon, Ford, Carter, Reagan, Bush, Clinton).

- You are in your car and think of four items you want from the grocery store and have no paper to write them on. You need butter, apples, lemon, and milk. By rearranging the first letters of these four items, you find that you can form the word "lamb," which will serve as a memory cue. If the items do not form a word, try making a sentence with matching first letters. For example, if your list is soup, chicken, soap, and lettuce, you could create the sentence "Some cooks like soup."

Additional Examples *(Group the First Letters of a Series of Items)*

Mr. Lewis, who lives in Utah, is reading a book that takes place in New England. He is uncertain which states are included in that geographical area, so he looks it up in the encyclopedia. He learns that the New England states include Maine, New Hampshire, Vermont, Connecticut, Massachusetts, and Rhode Island. He writes down the first letters of each state and works on creating a sentence whose words begin with the same letters as the six states, M-N-V-C-M-R. Mr. Lewis notes that the letters VCR stand for video cassette recorder and are already easily recalled as a group. He creates this sentence: "*Many VCR's Need Maintenance.*" Notice that, in this case, the order of the letters is not important.

EXERCISE: FIRST LETTER CUES

1. *Create a word or sentence out of the first letters of the names of these downtown streets to help you remember the order. In this case, it's important to keep the letters in the same order as the streets.*

   Main

   Adams

   Lincoln

   Rose

   Brown

   _____

   _____

   _____

   _____

2. *Try using this technique to remember the names of your cousin's children.*

   Rob

   Alice

   Chris

   _____

   _____

   _____

   _____

See p. 97 for possible solutions.

Expand Random Letters into a Familiar Word

Sometimes you need to remember a group of letters that make no inherent sense, for example, license plates or business names. In this case you can add more letters, often vowels, to form a familiar word.

EXAMPLES

- On a license plate, you might make the word "extra" out of "xra" or "lefty" out of "lft."

- If you have trouble remembering the name of the company that manages your apartment building, PND, expand these letters to form the word *panda*.

EXERCISE: CREATE A WORD

Expand the following letters into words:

1. PLM _____

2. RBT _____

3. GLW _____

4. STR _____

5. HLD _____

See p. 98 for possible solutions.

Group a List of Items by Category

Categorization is the process of looking at a random list of items and seeing how to group them by category. It is easier to remember three categories that serve as cues for the nine items in the list than to remember each of the nine items separately.

EXAMPLES

- The following nine items could be grouped into three categories:

popcorn	tuna	chips	applesauce	cookies
peas	milk	juice	pop	

Canned goods: peas applesauce tuna

Snacks: popcorn chips cookies

Liquids: milk juice pop

EXERCISE: CATEGORIZATION

Categorize the following items:

Windex	broom	paper towels
Scotch tape	envelopes	dish soap
glue	sponge	furniture polish
bleach		

_____

_____

_____

_____

_____

See p. 98 for possible solutions.

Additional Example *(Group a List of Items by Category)*

Imagine that you are trying to come up with a list of friends and acquaintances for an anniversary party. You might consider categories of friends, such as neighbors, work colleagues, church members, or card-playing friends. This technique would help you recall a larger number of your friends and acquaintances than would a random thought process.

Exercise for In-Class Use *(Are There Any Techniques That Could Help When I Have Several Items to Remember?)*

After you have taught the last five techniques, put a tray of twenty small items in an accessible place and ask students to study it during the coffee break. When you return to class, put the tray out of sight and ask students to list as many items as they can recall. After completing this assignment, ask students to discuss how they remembered the items. Note which techniques were used most frequently and which seemed most effective.

IS THERE ANYTHING THAT WILL HELP ME RECALL WELL-KNOWN INFORMATION WHEN I NEED IT?

When you know that the information you desire is in your long-term memory but you can't retrieve it when you want it, there are three techniques that you will find helpful:

- *Search your memory:* Search your memory bank for related facts that may serve as cues.
- *Alphabet search:* Go through the alphabet to jog your memory.
- *Review:* Review in advance what you may be called upon to remember.

Search Your Memory Bank for Related Facts That May Serve as Cues

When you can't think of something that you know is in your long-term memory, merely thinking longer and harder often does not work. However, there is a technique that is often useful. When you want to retrieve specific information from long-term memory, try thinking of related facts that serve as cues to trigger the information you are looking for.

This technique can be used for recalling:

- the name of a famous person
- the French word for *friend*
- the name of a TV show
- how to get somewhere that you haven't been for a long time
- the state in which the Grand Canyon is located.

┌─────── EXAMPLES ───────

- *Ms. Scott:* I met a woman at a party last week. When she introduced herself, I knew I had met her before. I remembered our interaction clearly, but I couldn't remember at whose home we had met. After I left the party, I searched for cues related to our initial meeting that would trigger the information about where we met. I thought about our conversation, how long ago the initial meeting took place, other people involved in the conversation, and my feelings about the interaction. It suddenly occurred to me that we had met earlier at a party given by a co-worker.

- *Mrs. McFadden:* My daughter lives in a new subdivision in town that has a special name, which I have trouble remembering. I wanted to tell my neighbor, but I didn't want to bother my daughter at work. I thought, "Maybe if I think of some related information, it will help." I could remember my daughter's address: 272 Appomattox. I thought about the entry sign to the subdivision that has a cannon on it. "It must have something to do with the Civil War." It came to me—Gettysburg!

EXERCISE: SEARCH YOUR MEMORY
See if you can recall the two candidates who ran for president of the United States in 1980. If you don't immediately know, search your memory for related facts that could serve as cues for this information.

_____

_____

See p. 98 for the answer.

Additional Example (*Search Your Memory Bank for Related Facts That May Serve as Cues*)

You are trying to remember the name of a favorite show from the early days of television. You think about the fact that it took place in the Old West, that the leading characters were a father and son, and that the father was played by Chuck Connors. You try to jog your memory by recalling the opening credits and whistling the theme song. You visualize the father as he appeared with a rifle in his hand, and it comes to you—"The Rifleman"!

Go through the Alphabet to Jog Your Memory

Alphabet search is the process of thinking through the sounds of the letters of the alphabet from *A* to *Z* to see if one will serve as a cue to jog your memory.

EXAMPLES

- If you're trying to remember the name of someone you have just met, run through the sounds of the alphabet. Hearing the sound of the letter *m* may trigger the name Marian.

- You want to describe the food you ate last night to a friend but can't remember the word *fettucine*. You might go through the alphabet hoping that the beginning sound of one of the letters will cue your memory.

Is there anything you can do to optimize your chances of remembering familiar names?

When you know in advance that you will be called upon to use the names of familiar persons, places, or things, you can use the following technique to prepare.

Review in Advance What You May Be Called upon to Remember

Everyone knows the feeling of forgetting familiar information, such as a friend's name or a well-known author. When you have to recall this type of information on demand, it sometimes takes a few seconds to bring it to mind—just long enough to cause a mental block. This experience is especially likely to happen if you are asked to recall something or someone you haven't thought about for a while. When you *know* you will be called upon to remember certain names or information, reviewing ahead of time will often eliminate this problem.

This technique can be used to help you keep in mind:

- the names of the grandnieces and grandnephews you will be seeing tomorrow
- the history of your medical problems when you see your doctor
- things you want to ask your grandchild when you take him out to lunch
- the names of people you will be seeing at the annual meeting of your condominium association

---

EXAMPLES

- If you are going to a family reunion or church social and are afraid you will not remember everyone's name, prepare ahead of time by going over a list of all who might attend. Writing down the names and saying them aloud is more effective than simply reading through a list. As you say the name, visualize the person and something special about him or her, like red hair or a great laugh.

- If you are going to a meeting of your book club, record the title of the book, the author, the names of characters, and your feelings about the book and review them before you go.

- If you are going to lunch with a friend, review the names of your friend's children and what you know about them beforehand so that you can talk about them easily.

Additional Examples *(Review in Advance What You May Be Called upon to Remember)*

You are volunteering in an elementary school tutoring three children in reading. They often tell you things about their families and assume that you will remember the facts when you see them again. For example, you learn that Jason has two sisters named Cecily and Leticia and a dog named Daisy. When he talks about Daisy, you would like to be sure that you remember who Daisy is. You decide to jot down facts about each child immediately after each tutoring session and review them before you see the child again.

Have you ever had the experience of going to a medical specialist and being unable to answer questions about the history of your problem? If you think ahead of time about what the doctor might ask you, you can reconstruct the history. Ask yourself when the symptoms began, when you saw your primary physician about this problem, and what treatments have been tried. Review the answers to these questions before you see the specialist so that you will be well prepared.

EXERCISE: REVIEW

Think of the next group meeting that you will attend (exercise class, senior center lunch group, bridge club, temple group) or try to think of the names of the people who live near you. List the names below and review them several times. If you have trouble listing all of them at one time, add to the list as the names come to you.

_____

_____

_____

_____

_____

_____

_____

_____

Did review help you remember the names more easily?

General Tips for Remembering

1. **Believe in yourself.** Don't let negative expectations defeat you. If you expect to fail, you won't even try. If you find yourself thinking, "I can't remember names," substitute "I may forget some names, but by using memory improvement techniques I can do better."

2. **Make conscious choices about what you want to remember.** No one can remember everything. So put effort and energy into those areas that are most important to you.

3. **Focus your attention on what you really want to remember.** Much of what is called forgetting is a lack of attention. Before you blame your memory, ask yourself if you were really paying attention.

4. **Cut out distractions.** Keep in mind that as you age, you may find it more difficult to pay attention to more than one thing at a time. Recognize the limitations of short-term memory and cut out distractions whenever possible.

5. **Give yourself plenty of time.** People of all ages forget more frequently when they are rushing. In general, if you have enough time to think about what you need to accomplish, you are less

likely to forget something. You may also find that you need more time for learning new information and for recalling information from long-term memory. Give yourself a little additional time and see if it helps in encoding and retrieving information.

6. **Use all of your senses.** Use as many senses as possible when you want to remember something well. When you say something aloud, you hear the sound. When you write something down, you see the words. If you want to remember the size or shape of something, use your sense of touch. Smell and taste are very powerful in triggering memories from long ago.

7. **Be organized.** The old saying, "A place for everything, and everything in its place" is good advice for memory improvement. Make a decision to improve your organizational skills in whatever ways are important to you. If you routinely put your keys, glasses, purse, and bills in the same place, you will not waste time searching for them.

8. **Recognize and deal with the factors that may be negatively affecting your memory.** Certain factors can affect the memory process for people of all ages, but as you grow older, you may experience more of these negative influences. Think about which factors might be affecting your memory and look for possible solutions or ways to compensate.

9. **Relax.** Tension interferes with the memory process; relaxing often lets the memory come to the surface. When you feel anxious about the possibility of forgetting, you may become preoccupied with the anxiety and unable to concentrate on recalling the needed information. The solution is to take a deep breath and relax; frequently the information will come to you.

10. **Laugh.** Laughter breaks the tension of forgetting and keeps a memory lapse in perspective. When you start to tell a friend about a book that you are reading and can't remember the title, or begin to introduce your niece and can't come up with her name, admit that the word or name just escaped your mind, and laugh. Everyone has had that experience and can empathize.

11. **Enjoy past memories.** Recognize the richness of your storehouse of memories. You can experience great pleasure from recalling the events and people that have made up the fabric of your life. Life review can put the past and present into perspective. Take pride in your ability to remember the past and make it come alive for yourself and others.

Answers to the Exercises

Recall (p. 10) **and Recognition** (p. 13)

1. Dogpatch
2. Judy Garland
3. Iwo Jima
4. Spiro Agnew

Understanding the Memory Process (pp. 14–15)

When you go to the library and notice that there are a lot of colorful books on the "new books" shelf, you are using *sensory memory*. You read through the titles and think about whether they interest you. These conscious thoughts occur in *short-term memory*. Then you notice a book by a favorite author, James Michener. You take down the book, notice how long it is, read the dust jacket, and decide that you don't have time to read it this month. This process is called *encoding*. The information about the book leaves your conscious thought and goes into *long-term memory*, where it may be available for *retrieval* at another time. When you get home, you notice another of Michener's books in your den. This favorite book serves as a *cue* and reminds you of the book in the library. The connection between the library book and your book is called *association*.

How Memory Works (p. 16)

1. F   5. T
2. F   6. T
3. T   7. F
4. T

Learning New Information (pp. 21–22)

1. Who and how many people you know
2. High motivation; low number of major life changes
3. Yes
4. It's important for older job seekers to get connected

How Memory Changes (p. 25)

1. F   4. T
2. F   5. F
3. T   6. T

Factors That Affect Memory (p. 50)

1. T   6. T
2. T   7. F
3. T   8. T
4. F   9. F
5. F   10. T

Association (p. 63)

1. Since you are going to the doctor, associate *west* with *wellness*.
2. Associate 1968 with the fact that the Tigers won the pennant that year, and you think of your grandson as a winner.
3. Associate *Campbell* with Campbell's soup and *Rose* with the red of the label on the soup can.
4. Associate the name *Turner* with turning your health around. Say to yourself several times, "Turner turned my health around."

Visualization (pp. 65–66)

1. Visualize a giant hammer hitting a man.
2. Imagine a tunnel with the sound of a heartbeat bouncing off the walls and echoing over and over.
3. Visualize a woman sitting in the park with the sun beating down on her shoulders.
4. Visualize five Balloons tied to your car antenna.
5. Visualize yourself paying for a tank of gas and asking the attendant for a replacement windshield wiper.

Environmental Change (pp. 74–75)

1. Put the pan in front of the door as soon as you think about bringing it.
2. Write yourself a note on the grocery bag in big letters so that when you unpack the groceries you'll see it.
3. Tie a string around your purse handle or wrist. When you get home you will be reminded to get the book out. Be sure to put it with your exercise clothes or equipment.
4. Put a big sign on the refrigerator or front door.
5. Change your watch or ring to the other hand.

Story Method (p. 79)

1. Envision a birthday cake shaped like a safe. You use a key to open it and find a huge pile of money.
2. See yourself breaking the bottle of cologne and sweeping up the pieces into a box of stationery.

First Letter Cues (p. 82)

1. Mother Always Liked Rose Best.
2. CAR or ARC

Create a Word (p. 83)

1. plum
2. robot
3. glow
4. string
5. hold

Categorization (p. 84)

Desk items	*Utensils*	*Cleaning products*
envelopes	sponge	Windex
Scotch tape	broom	dish soap
glue	paper towels	furniture polish
		bleach

Search Your Memory (p. 86)

Jimmy Carter and Ronald Reagan

Recommended Reading

Alan Baddeley. *Your Memory: A User's Guide*. New York: Macmillan, 1982.

Kathleen Gose and Gloria Levi. *Dealing with Memory Changes as You Grow Older*. New York: Bantam Books, 1988.

Danielle C. Lapp. *Don't Forget*. New York: McGraw-Hill, 1987.

Joan Minninger. *Total Recall*. New York: Pocket Books, 1984.

Edith Nalle Schafer. *Our Remarkable Memory*. Washington, D.C.: Starhill Press, 1988.

Robin West. *Memory Fitness over Forty*. Gainesville, Fla.: Triad Publications, 1985.

Review Exercises

The students have now learned sixteen memory improvement techniques. As they are presented with memory tasks, we hope they will have a repertoire of techniques to choose from that will be appropriate for the task and the situation. The following exercise can be used to stimulate discussion about possible solutions to some common memory challenges.

How Do I Remember to Do Something That Needs to Be Done in the Future?

Basic task: Set up a cue that will remind you when the time comes.

Task examples:
take something with you when you go somewhere
pick up something when you are out
make a phone call
turn off your car lights when you reach your destination

Possible techniques:
auditory reminder
written reminder
environmental change

Scenario: You need to call your daughter when she gets home from work to tell her that you cannot babysit for her next weekend. She is a teacher and you cannot call her at work. She will be home from work in two hours—at 5:00.

Possible solutions:
Set the alarm clock for two hours.
Write a note and put it in on the TV, because you always watch the 5:00 news.
Put the phone on the floor in front of the TV instead of in its usual place.

How Can I Be Sure to Remember Something I Have Recently Done?

Basic task: Paying attention and encoding information so that you can remember what you have done in the recent past.

Task examples:
where you put your glasses, keys, shoes
where you parked your car
whether you have taken your medications
where you hid something

Possible techniques:
written reminder
association
active observation
self-instruction
organization

Scenario: You are going on a trip for a month. There have recently been break-ins in your community. You decide to hide your jewelry in the linen closet in the bathroom, but you know that in the past you have forgotten a hiding place when you have been gone for so long.

Possible solutions:
Make a note of the hiding place on your calendar for the day of your return.
Use association: I hid my *jewelry* in the *john*.
Actively observe yourself hiding the jewelry, and imagine how a burglar might search for it.
Say to yourself aloud, "I hid my jewelry in the linen closet where no burglar will ever find it."
Be organized. Always use the same hiding place.

How Can I Avoid Forgetting Something When I Have Several Things to Do?

Basic task: Connecting the information so that you have just one thing to remember that will trigger a memory of the rest.

Task examples: grocery items
jobs to do
errands to run
names

Possible techniques: story method
group first letters
visualization
written reminder

Scenario: You have three errands to do—go to the post office, pick up cleaning, and go to the bank. In the past you have gotten home only to realize that you forgot to do one of the errands. You want to be able to keep them all in mind.

Possible solutions: Make up a story that you went to the post office, put the purchased stamps in your coat pocket, then left the coat to be cleaned and ruined the stamps, making it necessary for you to go to the bank to get money for more stamps.
Use the first letter of each destination to make one word or set of initials that you can remember: Post office = P; Cleaners = C; Bank = B. PCB is the name of chemical poison with which you may be familiar.
Visualize the route you take between the post office, cleaners, and bank.
Write a list of the errands and tape it to your dashboard.

How Can I Recall Something When It Is on the "Tip of My Tongue"?

Basic task: Retrieving something from long-term memory into short-term memory (or conscious thought).

Task examples: names of people
titles of books, TV shows, movies
names of places

Possible techniques: mental retracing
alphabet search
relax and think of something else; the information may surface

Scenario: You want to call and make a reservation at a new restaurant that is not yet listed in the yellow pages, but you can't remember its name.

Possible solutions: Begin thinking of other related information: the street it is on; some nearby stores; the friend who first mentioned it; and the kind of food served. One of these facts may trigger recall of the forgotten information.
Say the letters of the alphabet slowly. First letters are often very good cues.
Go read the newspaper. When you are relaxed, forgotten information often comes to mind.

**How Can I Remember What I've Seen, Read, and Heard So That
I Can Repeat It Later?**

Basic task: Paying attention and storing information effectively so that it can be recalled at a future time.

Task examples: conversations
information from newspapers, books
information from radio, TV, movies
name of a new person

Possible techniques: association and visualization
active observation
written reminder

Scenario: You hear some interesting new information on the radio about foods that seem to prevent cancer. You want to tell your friend what you have heard.

Possible solutions: Envision a big salad with all of the food items in it. Associate them with one another.
Actively think about the food items, asking yourself if you like them, how frequently you eat them, whether your friend likes them.
Write down the food items so that you can refer to the note when you talk to your friend.

How to Offer a Memory Course

A memory course based on the materials in this book can be offered in four consecutive weekly sessions of two hours each, although more sessions can be added if desired. This course is designed for people who are experiencing the normal changes in memory that occur with age, not for those who have dementia. The objectives of the course are:

1. to challenge the belief held by many older adults that they have little control over their ability to improve memory;
2. to provide information that will help each participant understand his or her own memory functioning and learn ways to improve it;
3. to alleviate anxiety about memory changes through information and examples;
4. to provide a safe and comfortable atmosphere that will allow participants to discuss their present and future concerns regarding both memory and aging;
5. to create an environment where participants can see the humorous side of forgetting and laugh with others as they share experiences;
6. to provide information on topics related to memory, such as nutrition, medication awareness, and stress; and
7. to reinforce the idea that late life can be a time of learning and continued growth.

Publicity

You will probably find that there is a lot of interest in memory improvement among older adults in your community. However, initially you may need to publicize your course widely. Below are some of the means that we have found effective.

1. News releases are mailed out at least one month before the course begins. The releases are sent to newspapers, radio stations, religious organizations, and community agencies. These organizations are usually willing to incorporate the information into their bulletins. Sometimes the bulletins are aimed at the older population, but, whatever the case, people who hear or see the announcement will help spread the word to other people who might want to participate.
2. Flyers are mailed to senior centers, public agencies, religious organizations, doctors' offices, businesses, senior housing complexes, service providers, and anyone else who might post them on their bulletin boards. (See the sample flyer on p. 100.)
3. The same flyers or informative letters announcing the memory programs are sent to individuals who have participated in other, similar, activities. The agency offering the course (senior center, YMCA, and so on) can usually provide a mailing list composed of potentially interested people.
4. The memory course is also publicized whenever program leaders give short talks to groups of seniors (church circles, for example) or consult with individuals by telephone who have concerns about their memory skills.
5. After the program has been established, new participants are usually easily recruited through word-of-mouth recommendations from satisfied participants.

Membership

We ask potential participants to register by telephone. During the phone conversation, we make an effort to explore whether the participant's objectives can be met within the framework of the course. We are reluctant to enroll any memory-impaired people who may be unable to follow the content of the course, and we do not offer hope for improvement of severe memory problems. Occasionally a person calls with concerns about the

IMPROVING YOUR MEMORY

A Course for Older Adults

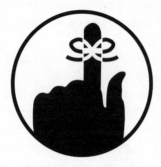

Would you like to learn more about:

How memory works
How memory changes with age
Factors that can cause changes in memory
Techniques for improving memory

University of Michigan Medical Center's
Turner Geriatric Services
1010 Wall Street

Four sessions will be held on consecutive Thursdays.
March 26, April 2, April 9, and April 16
from 1:30 to 3:30 P.M.

Fee for the course is $20 plus the cost of the text.
Preregistration is required.

very real memory problems of his or her partner. It may be beneficial to accept such a couple even if one spouse is memory-impaired, because the caller will gain understanding about normal changes in memory from the content of the course.

Even though we attempt to screen out inappropriate participants over the telephone, the composition of the group is often varied in terms of the cognitive skills of the members. We have found that diversity in abilities is not an insurmountable problem, because group members are generally very understanding of differences and supportive of one another's concerns. During telephone screening, participants are told that attendance at all sessions is required, because the course material of each session will build on the material in the preceding one.

Registration is limited to between fifteen and twenty people, because an important part of the course involves individual participation and group interaction. If the cut-off number for registration is reached, a waiting list can be established for the next offering of the course.

Confidentiality

The establishment of confidentiality and trust among the participants, as well as nonjudgmental acceptance of the concerns and problems of others, is essential. The leader can state that in order for everyone to get the most out of the course, participants should feel free to discuss their problems without worrying about whether their stories will be repeated elsewhere. This understanding is especially important in a small community, where people are likely to share social acquaintances.

Fees

After several years of offering this course free as a service to the community, we discovered that people are quite willing to pay a fee and may put in more effort because of their investment. We charge five dollars for each session plus the cost of *Improving Your Memory: How to Remember What You're Starting to Forget.* Scholarships are always available for those who have financial limitations.

Leadership

Over the years, a variety of people have led our memory courses: professional staff, including social workers, nurses, and educators; nursing and social work students; and peer counselors. Leaders must have knowledge about memory and aging, as well as about group process.

Our course model is based on shared leadership, with two leaders taking turns presenting various aspects of the course material. Having the regularly scheduled opportunity to sit back and observe group participation and interaction, without being responsible for presenting material, allows the leaders to assess the impact of the course and the needs of participants. Also, there are always participants who want to have questions answered individually or who desire confidential consultation, and two leaders are twice as accessible during the break and at the meeting's end. Although we have found co-leadership to be valuable, this is not to say that a single leader can't present a successful program.

It's very important for the leaders to maintain a certain amount of flexibility regarding the course content, as well as to vary the content to fit the needs and interests of the participants. If there are people in the class who have significant memory deficits, the material or the pace of the course can be altered, and certain exercises that might prove too frustrating can be omitted.

Over the years, we have discovered the importance of the following concepts:

1. Humor is a vital part of the memory course. Participants love sharing funny stories about how they have forgotten things. Laughter can take the sting out of embarrassing moments and create a feeling of connection among the participants. These stories also illustrate that everyone forgets something from time to time. People especially enjoy hearing about the leaders' memory slips, and these should be admitted freely.

2. Goal setting is essential to memory improvement. To help participants recognize that improvement has occurred, they should be instructed to set very specific goals and monitor their progress. For example, if Bob's goal is to stop misplacing his keys

and he finds ways to achieve this goal, he will feel successful and will be encouraged to tackle other problems.

3. Leaders should find a way to help everyone in the class feel successful. To accomplish this, some exercises must be included that will allow all participants to succeed. Leaders must also ask for and validate participants' creative solutions.

4. The more habitually the leaders employ memory techniques in their own lives, the better they will understand the memory process and the more enthusiastic they will be about the material.

Set Up

If possible, participants should be seated at tables so that they can easily take notes and perform in-class exercises. We arrange the tables so that participants face one another. This encourages group interaction and support and makes it easier for everyone to hear other participants. We make name plates out of folded pieces of paper with first and last names in large print on both front and back. The participants stand their name plates on the table in front of them, place-card style, so that they can be easily seen by all. The name plates allow us to proceed on a first-name basis without embarrassment over forgotten names, although one of the assignments of the memory course will be to learn one another's names.

Each participant receives an inexpensive folder with pockets, which contains a copy of *Improving Your Memory,* the list of participants' names, and some blank paper for note-taking. Remembering to bring the folder to each session can be considered one memory assignment.

Throughout the course, we make use of the practice of going around the table asking each person to briefly respond to a question or topic of discussion so that everyone has an opportunity to contribute. This routine, yet nonthreatening, responsibility to the discussion format enables even the shyer members to feel comfortable taking part in the group discussion. However, we never put pressure on people to respond, and they have the option of passing on any go-around. Also, regular opportunity for participant-initiated questions and discussion should be given by the leader. Many participants are reluctant to interrupt if they don't understand something, yet need clarification, or need to have material repeated.

We take a break of between ten and fifteen minutes in the middle of the two-hour session. Coffee and tea are always available, and we provide cookies for the first session. Volunteers bring cookies to the next three sessions.

Homework

At the beginning of the course, participants are told that they will be given homework assignments to practice what they are learning. We have found that active participation in class and an integration of the material into daily life greatly enhances the potential for change.

Evaluation

Over the years our program has changed based on input from the participants. We recommend both the anonymity of a written evaluation form at the end of the course and ongoing interactive group discussion as ways to elicit information on the effectiveness of the program as a whole and of its individual parts.

Memory Course Evaluation

In order to make the memory course as useful as possible, we would like your comments. We rely on them to make changes that will improve future courses. Thank you.

1. The program gave me new information.   Agree   Disagree

2. The information was practical to me.   Agree   Disagree

3. I will use one of the techniques taught to improve my memory.   Agree   Disagree

4. The time allowed for discussion and questions was sufficient.   Agree   Disagree

5. The discussion relieved some of my anxiety about memory changes.   Agree   Disagree

6. I would like more information on _____

7. How did you learn about this course? Check as many as apply.

    ( ) Family   ( ) Doctor

    ( ) Friend   ( ) Newspaper; which one? _____

    ( ) Flyer   ( ) Other _____

8. How can we improve this course?

9. How was this course helpful to you?

Sample Agenda for a Four-Session Memory Course

Time required for each session: two hours, including a ten- to fifteen-minute break.

Session One

1. Have participants introduce themselves and state why they chose to attend a memory course.

2. Ask participants how many names they can recall from the introductions, excluding those that they already know. You can expect that most participants will remember very few names.

3. Discuss the difficulty in remembering names due to the following facts:

   Names have little inherent meaning.

   We often pay little attention to the name when we are introduced to someone.

   We rarely give adequate thought to how to remember names.

4. Reintroduce yourself and describe an effective method of giving meaning to your name. Provide visual associations for your name with a simple sketch. (For examples, see opposite.)

Hand out blank paper and bold magic markers and instruct participants to draw pictures that represent a visual association for their own names. If anyone has trouble with this exercise, you or other participants can help think of a good association. Have each participant display his or her picture and explain the association. Ask people again how many names they can recall from these introductions. Usually, participants can remember many more names this time around. If a copy machine is readily available, make copies of each drawing at the break, and give them to participants for home study in between sessions. If not, have participants take notes on the names and their visual associations for review between sessions.

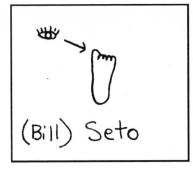

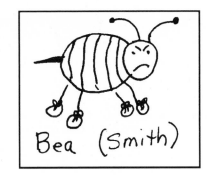

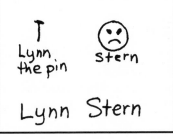

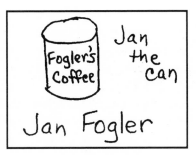

5. Hand out name plates.

6. Present details of what to expect from the course and information on the physical setting and group procedures:

   - breaks at every session
   - refreshments if desired and volunteers to bring them
   - location of rest rooms
   - confidentiality
   - collection of fees
   - attendance and commitment
   - homework at each session

7. Present information on how memory works (see pp. 3–17).

8. Teach three techniques: association, visualization, and active observation (see pp. 64–68).

9. Homework assignments:

   - Monitor one situation in which you are apt to be forgetful, and observe successes and failures in trying to remember. It's important to limit this task to a very specific behavior or situation; for example, keeping track of a medication regimen, remembering where you put your keys or glasses, or learning the names of people in your exercise class. Keep a record of this assignment and, when memory lapses do occur, write down the circumstances.
   - Learn fellow participants' names by reviewing the list of names or the photocopied set of drawings.
   - Read the portions in the text on how memory works and the three techniques presented today. Do all accompanying exercises.

10. Present a brief preview of next session.

Session Two

1. Before handing out the name plates, ask if anyone would like to try to name all of the participants. (Usually, someone will have worked hard on this assignment and will welcome the opportunity to try.) If not, ask the group collectively to name as many participants as they can. Usually, some portion of each name can be recalled. This exercise generally creates a feeling of success and demonstrates that it is possible to learn a group of new names using association and visualization as effective techniques.

2. Hand out name plates.

3. Have participants report on homework assignments.

4. Briefly review the information on how memory works.

5. Present information on how memory changes with age and the first six factors that affect memory (see pp. 19–27).

6. Teach four techniques: mental elaboration, written reminders, auditory reminders, and environmental change (see pp. 69–75).

7. Homework assignments:

   - Read the portions in the text on how memory changes with age, the first six factors that affect memory, and the four techniques presented today. Do the accompanying exercises.
   - Choose two techniques from the seven presented in the last two sessions and try them in daily life. Write down successes and failures.
   - Using the technique of active observation, choose something of interest to observe in detail each day, for example, the view outside your window, the antics of your pet, or the set of your favorite TV show. Look at familiar objects with a fresh eye. Note any new observations about familiar scenes.

8. Present a brief preview of next session.

Session Three

1. Have volunteers pick a name plate from the pile and give it to the correct person.

2. Hand out the remaining name plates.

3. Have participants report on homework assignments.

4. Briefly review how memory changes with age.

5. Teach remaining eight factors that affect memory and six techniques: self-instruction, story method, chunking, group first letters, create a word, and categorization (see pp. 76–84).

6. Homework assignments:
   • Read the portions in the text on the last eight factors that affect memory and the six techniques presented today. Do accompanying exercises.
   • Choose two techniques from all presented and use them in daily life. Monitor successes and failures.

7. Present a brief preview of next session.

Session Four

1. Ask if anyone wants to try to remember as many names as she or he can. Give anyone who wants to try a chance.

2. Hand out name plates.

3. Ask participants to report on homework.

4. Teach three techniques: search your memory bank, alphabet search, and review in advance.

5. Present the scenarios from the review exercise on pp. 95–97 and have participants consider various techniques that could be used to perform the memory tasks. Ask participants if they have any unresolved memory problems that the group could help them solve.

6. Ask participants to discuss ways that they will work on improving memory in the future.

7. Present summary of highlights of the course.

8. Collect participant evaluation. (This can be handed out during the break. See p. 102.)

Recommended Reading

Alan Baddeley. *Your Memory: A User's Guide.* New York: Macmillan, 1982.

Alan S. Brown. *How to Increase Your Memory Power.* Glenview, Ill.: Scott Foresman, 1989.

Kathleen Gose and Gloria Levi. *Dealing with Memory Changes as You Grow Older.* New York: Bantam Books, 1988.

Danielle C. Lapp. *Don't Forget.* New York: McGraw-Hill, 1987.

_____. *Maximizing Your Memory Power.* Hauppauge, N.Y.: Barron's Educational Series, 1992.

Elizabeth Loftus. *Memory.* Reading, Mass.: Addison-Wesley, 1982.

Joan Minninger. *Total Recall.* New York: Pocket Books, 1984.

Leonard W. Poon et al., eds. *Everyday Cognition in Adulthood and Late Life.* Cambridge: Cambridge University Press, 1989.

Edith Nalle Schafer. *Our Remarkable Memory.* Washington, D.C.: Starhill Press, 1988.

Robin West. *Memory Fitness over Forty.* Gainesville, Fla.: Triad Publications, 1985.

Notes:

Notes:

Notes:

Notes:

Notes:

Notes:

Notes:

Notes:

Library of Congress Cataloging-in-Publication Data
Folger, Janet.
  Teaching memory improvement to adults / Janet Fogler and Lynn Stern.—Rev. ed.
      p.   cm.
  Includes bibliographical references.
  ISBN 0-8018-4769-9 (pbk. : alk. paper)
  1. Memory in old age—Study and teaching.   2. Memory—Age factors—Study and
teaching.   3. Mnemonics—Study and teaching.   I. Stern, Lynn, 1949–   .   II. Title
BF724.85.M45F66   1994
153.1'2'-0846—dc20   93-36784